Our Secret Super Power

Harness the Power of the Mind to Live a Healthier and Happier Life

Ranjeev Singh Sidhu MRPharmS

"The mind is a powerful thing though this is often overlooked when treatment options are discussed. A good read for all patients and healthcare professionals."

Janice Perkins - Chair RPS Community Pharmacy Expert Advisory Group

This book tackles a subject with the potential to disrupt modern life's expectations of guaranteed quick fixes offered, misplaced, in traditional medicines. The author alerts us to the potential of placebo's as a valid alternative - and as a Healthcare Digital Leader - this book excited me with the opportunities that emerging Patient Health Records offer to capture the everyday placebo evidence via a patient's own recording.

Phill James - Digital Clinical System Programme Director at Mid Cheshire Hospitals NHS Foundation Trust & East Cheshire NHS Trust

"An undeniably powerful and human perspective on healthcare that can sometimes be lost in modern medicine. These touching stories provide striking evidence for the power of the most researched medicine in the world — the placebo effect. Not only does this book illustrate its versatility in both health and disease it also poignantly shows its ubiquitous nature — we all have access to it, we need only unlock its potential."

India Pinker — Medical Education, University of St Andrews

RANJEEV SINGH SIDHU

Our Secret Super Power
Published by Psy-Qi Ltd
16 Jubilee Parkway
Derby

Copyright © 2022 Ranjeev Singh Sidhu
Book design and illustrations by ArtCore, Derby

All rights reserved. No part of this book may be reproduced, scanned or distributed in any printed or electronic format without permission.

ISBN

Disclaimer

This book provides general information and discussions about health and related subjects. The information and other content provided in this book, or in any linked materials, are not intended and should not be construed as medical advice, nor is the information a substitute for professional medical expertise or treatment. If you or any other person has a medical concern, you should consult with your health care provider or seek other professional medical treatment.

Never disregard professional medical advice or delay in seeking it because of something that you have read in this book or in any linked materials. If you think you may have a medical emergency, call your doctor or emergency services immediately. The opinions and views expressed on this book and website have no relation to those of any academic, hospital, health practice or other institution.

When highlighting the shortcomings of Big Pharma or modern approaches to medicine, the purpose is not to discredit the profession but to encourage a more holistic approach to healthcare that puts the patient at the heart of their own health development. The intention is to add the art of healing to the science of medicine.

All names in the case studies have been changed to protect the privacy of the individuals involved.

About the Author

I'm a qualified pharmacist who has spent over 20 years investigating the health industry to understand more about how and why we treat patients as we do.

As well as being a qualified pharmacist, having worked in and managed my own independent pharmacy, I'm also a highly sought-after executive coach (ILM7 senior exec coach). Today I work with several UK-listed companies to support and develop the way they manage and think about their businesses.

My first book, *Sai: A Spiritual Journey*, was hugely celebrated in India, launched by the Vice President, and was even presented to Shehbaz Sharif, the current president of Pakistan, as a gift. It was a big honour for me.

I'm proud to work with The Prince's Trust as a mentor for young people and I feel honoured to be participating in the 'Beyond Pills' steering group (A campaign that was launched summer 2022 at the House of Lords).

If you would like to speak to me about anything in this book, or would like to book a wellbeing consultation for you or your organisation, feel free to email me

enquiries@psy-qi.com

Contents

Preface   11

Foreword   15

Acknowledgements   17

Introduction: 19
How A Rookie Mistake Changed Angela's Life (And Mine)

Chapter One: 35
Your Body Is An Incredible Piece Of Kit

Chapter Two: 51
What Is The Placebo Effect?

Chapter Three: 69
How The Placebo Effect Became So Misunderstood

Chapter Four: 83
Health Is An Inside Job

Chapter Five: 99
Pushback And Politics

Chapter 6:   113
A Better Way For Everyone

Chapter Seven: 125

There's Nothing Stopping You From Evolving

Conclusion: 137
How The Placebo Effect Can Help You Take
Control Of Your Own Health

Highlights From The Research 157

Further Reading 161

Preface

What this book is about
Our Superpower is about giving you the tools and insight you need to live a healthier and happier life.

Though that might sound like a humble aim, the truth is, in sharing how you can recreate the mental and *physical* impact of what's known as 'the placebo effect,' my intention with this book is to cause a complete revolution in your thinking and way of life.

Be clear, *Our Secret Superpower* is not a book solely *about* the placebo effect per se, nor is it a book designed to merely *prove* the existence of the phenomenon. This book is about establishing how the *impact* of what is commonly called the placebo effect is of much greater importance to our well-being, both mental and physical, than many of us realise. But in doing so, I face a fundamental challenge.

The word 'placebo' and the ideas associated with it have become a modern cliché. Often, we use the term in a dismissive, negative way: *Oh, it's just a placebo*. This is wrong. In my experience as a qualified pharmacist, and as this book looks to evidence, the true impact of what we dismiss as 'placebo' can be life changing. It can turn hopeless situations into hopeful ones, dire prognosis into transformational opportunities.

As I say, this book is about how you can understand, harness and recreate the real-world impact of a placebo if you are experiencing poor health outcomes of any kind. In other words, harness the *power* of the placebo effect, a secret superpower we all have inside.

In examining what the placebo effect is, how it works, and *why* it works, and by sharing with you real-world examples of it in action, this book aims to not only breakdown the misconceptions about how we perceive the placebo effect but provide a new and original framework for harnessing and recreating the real-world impact it can have on our lives.

Make no mistake, *Our Secret Superpower* is about changing your life, and about how to harness the power that you already have inside you.

Who this book is for

First and foremost, *Our Secret Superpower* is for anyone who wants to seek a happier and healthier way of living.

Though I'm convinced the ideas in this book will help those who are, this is not just a book for anyone who might currently be living with a medical health condition. It is for anyone and everyone who has a feeling that there might be a better way to live, for anyone and everyone who has already realised that carrying the stresses of modern life on their shoulders twenty-four seven is not healthy.

It is also a book for those who are curious, those who doubtful and those who are fed-up, having tried everything to 'get better' but cannot seem to find any answers. Though I don't claim to have all the answers, I hope this book will act as a springboard to help you find the ones that you are looking for.

How this book is structured
You'll see this is a short and simple book. It is not intended to be a complicated 'science book' or an academic text.

It is written in such a way as to make it possible for you to read it easily and quickly. It is broken down into seven short chapters. Each chapter can be read in one sitting and, as you move through the book, you will see that I aim to first explain what the placebo effect is, why it's so useful, and why it has become so misunderstood. From there, I'll show you how you can harness its power for yourself using very simple techniques.

Once you've read the whole of *Our Secret Superpower*, I hope you'll be able to return time and time again to help remind yourself of the simple techniques you can put in practice in your daily routine to ultimately transform your health and life.

13

Foreword

This is not just a good book, it is a great book and also a very important one.

The placebo effect is the most powerful comprehensive medicine that we have as doctors and sadly neglected in the health service, where continuing care, compassion and relationships are continually downgraded as priorities. That is why this book is so important. It casts a new light on the placebo effect and that much needed change in perspective. It is supported by some excellent advice on how we can improve self-healing in our own lives as an area that all of us should seek to explore.

Indeed, this is a book for everyone and in just a few pages it has the potential to change both the length and the quality of life for so many of us.

In short, Ranjeev Sidhu offers us a key to unlocking our sick and weary lives and restoring the power to heal ourselves.

By Dr Michael Dixon LVO, OBE, MA, FRCGP

Former Chair of NHS Alliance & President of the NHS Clinical Commissioners

Acknowledgements

Firstly, I'd like to convey my gratitude to Pam for her commitment to this project and helping to bring it into the world. It has been a long difficult journey made a little easier with her by my side.

I am deeply thankful to Prof Dave Gerrett, my PhD supervisor, and Dr Michael Dixon, who was able to, as far back as 2001, see the big picture and help me to draw out the essence of the placebo effect at a time when there was little interest in this field.

I am also thankful to Anna Farley, lead researcher for this book, for her vital part in transforming my ideas into a manuscript that is now in a format that can be understood by medical and non-medical people, alike. Also, to Glenn Fisher who helped to structure the book and the editing to create this wonderful, finished piece of work.

I would also like to extend my gratitude to Dr Michael Dixon, Janice Perkins, Phill James, Sarah Ball, India Pinker and Luci Devenport who were kind enough to review and provide helpful feedback and additional input.

Finally, I would like to express my love for all those who have supported the project over the past 20 years, either financially, emotionally or practically.

Thank you from the bottom of my heart.

Introduction:

How A Rookie Error Changed Angela's Life (And Mine)

'What lies behind us and what lies before us are tiny matters compared to what lies within us'
— Ralph Waldo Emerson

Angela was an advanced stage cancer patient. And when she came into the pharmacy, I could tell she was clearly in a lot of pain.

Her prescription confirmed my thoughts. It was for Fentanyl, a painkiller estimated to be up to one hundred times more powerful than morphine. Just two milligrams (less than four grains of sugar) can kill. She took the drug through patches that stuck to her skin, constantly releasing small amounts of Fentanyl into her body in a safe and controlled manner.

When Angela walked in, it was 1999 and I'd only just landed my first job as a pharmacist manager. With my brand-new degree, I'd landed the job at a little pharmacy in Altrincham. I'd been training for years and now I finally had the chance to really make people's lives better. It was good pharmacy job: giving advice, managing the pharmacy, dispensing medicines. I was extremely happy.

However, just three months into the job, I had an experience that dramatically changed my thinking and the trajectory of my life. It was insignificant in the bigger scheme of things, but had such an impact on my thinking that it played on my mind and does so even to this day. What exactly happened here?

Angela was in the pharmacy, and she was furious. She had every reason to be angry, the medication that she ordered failed to arrive. I felt terrible for the oversight: leaving a cancer patient with no pain medication was the last thing I wanted to do.

After I apologised profusely, she told me that she would need the patch for the following evening as that's when she was due to change it. A sigh of relief that we had some time, I reordered the Fentanyl right there and then, promising to have it for her by the following morning.

The next day, the pharmacy opened at eight thirty sharp and there was Angela. My heart sank when she came in. A panic set in. Had I ordered the medicine? Did I send the order? Yes, and yes, I thought. But I walked over, and she wasn't happy that the Fentanyl patches still weren't there.

"You said it would be here in the morning," she said.

Feeling worse than ever, I sheepishly explained that by 'next morning' I meant 'some time before twelve'. I realised I needed to be clearer in my communication in the future. Deliveries arrived just before ten.

To save her coming back to the pharmacy again, I offered to deliver the medicine to her that evening. At five thirty I left work and headed over to her house, not wanting to keep her waiting any longer. I knocked on the door. No answer. I knocked again just in case. Nothing. I kept knocking and knocking but still no reply.

At that point, I was pretty much stuck. There I was, standing on the street, holding a bag of controlled drugs. I certainly couldn't take them back home with me, and I couldn't take them to the pharmacy either, since that was closed and, until I had a signature from her, I couldn't leave them. There are legal restrictions.

I waited for around half an hour or so, knocking and knocking, thinking maybe she'd gone out. Just as I was really giving up she answered the door.

She was in a dressing gown, hair dripping wet, and if I thought she'd been angry before it was nothing compared to this. She was very upset, shouting at me on the street.

"I've been waiting all day and you came when I was in the shower!" she snapped.

All I could do was hand over the medicine and apologise. I got the signature and walked away with my tail between my legs. I'd only been in the job for three months, and I'd already had my first major challenge.

The next day Angela was back in the pharmacy again. I was too scared to face her. I tried to get someone else to deal with it, but she insisted she wanted to speak to me. I couldn't even look at her.

To my complete surprise, as soon as she set eyes on me, she *didn't* start yelling again. There was a difference in her demeanour, but I couldn't quite put my finger on it.

"Look," she said, "I am sorry about yesterday and I really wanted to thank you for coming around last night."

"No, no," I reassured her, assuming she was trying to apologise for shouting, "It was my mistake and delivering the medicines was no bother at all."

"No, you don't understand," Angela said. "After you left, I sat down on the sofa, and I fell asleep. I didn't end up putting the patch on last night and I had the best sleep I've had in months."

I didn't know what to say. A good sleep, the best she'd had in years? A seemingly normal event for most people but those of you who have experienced this kind of pain, you'll know it really isn't that normal. The day before, Angela had been so convinced she needed the Fentanyl patches, she felt she could not go a moment without them. And yet, not only had she not used it, apparently, for some reason, she had a really good deep sleep.

When I finally got the courage to meet her eyes, I realised that she looked different. She looked fresh, natural, so much more full of life compared to the person who came in just a day ago.

I had no idea what had prompted the change. I was under no illusion that this was permanent but there was no doubt that something had happened. It wasn't the drugs. It wasn't me. And I don't know of any other influencing factor.

Whatever happened to Angela, had happened *inside* her.

The change was profound, and I couldn't understand it. Clearly, something had happened, I didn't really know what. Was it something to do with being angry at me and releasing some deep-rooted pain? Was it a mindset shift? Instead of thinking about her illness, was it because she had something else to focus on, Or maybe it was a combination of other factors? I didn't know. But I was intrigued.

This was something my pharmaceutical training hadn't prepared me for. But it had lit a fire in me.

Indeed, my experience with Angela reminded me of my own past. As a child, I had a skin condition called Ichthyosis. My skin would get so dry, peel and shed like the skin of a snake. I couldn't sweat either. On a hot day I'd turn bright red, and my skin would expand like a balloon as there was no way for the heat to escape. In the UK, we tried everything, all the standard treatments the doctors could offer: topical steroids, all types of weird and wonderful creams and shampoos. I was in the Children's Hospital regularly. But none of the treatments really made much of a difference to my condition. Yes, my skin was less dry after applying the creams, but it very quickly turned even drier than before.

Eventually, when I was twelve years old, my family went to India. We were advised to try the hot volcanic sulphur waters in the Himalayas. At the foot of the Himalayas there was a place called Manali, in the amazing Kullu valley. Picture postcard stuff. It took us a couple of days to get there. Just the scenery made the trip worthwhile. We were advised to bathe twice a day and see what happened.

The water was hot, very hot, and I had to sit for fifteen to twenty minutes at a time. But then something incredible happened. I started to sweat. And I've been able to sweat since then. I wasn't completely cured but my condition improved. The change was significant and tangible. As a result of being able to sweat, I could run further and faster, and participate better at school games.

Western medicine had a lot of answers, but it certainly didn't have all the answers. Not for Angela and not for me. This feeling I got when I thought about these rare and strange occurrences was profound and led me to conclude that my education wasn't complete. I quit within a few months of getting my first job, setting aside the career I'd worked so hard for to find answers.

My parents, first generation immigrants, were puzzled: "Why are you leaving such a good job? Do a couple more years, get some money in the bank, buy a house, and then you can do what you like."

But I knew, and they knew, that I had made up my mind. This was too important to me. Luckily, they were supportive of my decision.

I started on this new journey. I received formal training as a natural medicine pharmacist. I studied Anthroposophical Medicine, Hypnotherapy, Acupuncture, Homeopathy, Ayurvedic medicine, everything, and anything I could get my hands on. I even started a PhD.

And the one thing I kept running into again and again as I studied all these alternative and complementary medicines was the vital role a patient's mind and lifestyle plays in their health status. It was then I stumbled across something that was present in both western and complementary approaches to medicine.

It was my first Ah-ha moment:

The Placebo Effect.

Was the placebo effect responsible for many of the transformational events that I had read and witnessed? We had studied it at university but never in this context or in any detail.

I remember I used to get annoyed when some of the academic experts would snigger at any form of non-western therapy, dismissing it as, *'Oh, that's just the placebo effect.'* I realise now that I was very naïve about the economics of health and why these opinions came about.

Later I was to learn that there are very real reasons why medical professional think the way they think. There just isn't enough money to be made by making people better.

From a pharmaceutical industry point of view, a patient healed is a customer lost. Not only that, but accepting that complementary medicine does work would 'force' them to re-evaluate their purely scientific worldview.

As you likely know, the placebo effect is the most researched procedure in all of medicine. Yet there is a disconnect here.

We know that the placebo effect is used extensively in clinical trials as the 'gold standard' that new drugs need to beat to get approval, yet we totally disregard it in the community setting.

In these trials, some patients are given a placebo treatment – such as a sugar pill, or an injection containing saline – and surprisingly there is a marked improvement, despite not receiving a real drug.

These observations aren't rare either. No, the placebo effect shows up so often that it has been the standard that all drugs have to beat to get the coveted and lucrative medicinal license. Ironically enough, because of this, placebos have a habit of getting a bad reputation.

A leading researcher from Stanford University explains the problem extremely well. If a drug passes 'the placebo test' the drug is a success and will go on to be licensed, whereas the placebo is side-lined and of no more use. But if the drug doesn't beat the placebo. The placebo is seen as the villain, the cause of billions of pounds being wasted.

Whether a drug passes clinical trial, or not, the placebo has never been given the respect it deserves. Just think of how many times you have heard a person who responds positively to some treatment that they later find out has no scientific evidence.

Placebo, I came to learn, is not 'just the placebo' but is a vital component of the healing process. It has also been suggested that the placebo effect triggers the healing effect. This is incredible. In this context, the placebo effect is solid proof of the body's ability to heal itself.

Placebo means 'I shall please' in Latin. But I wasn't just pleased, I was fascinated. The research in this field had captured my imagination and now over 20 years later, I am even more convinced that understanding and harnessing the power of the placebo effect is a key part of solving the health crisis we face in the 21st century.

Yet the irony is that as a healthcare professional I am not allowed to give a placebo, it is seen as deceptive and has many ethical issues.

Whether the alternative therapies I studied, or the new drugs under research, have any powers of their own or not, one thing is for sure, they all tapped into and harnessed this powerful healing force, what I like to call your innate superpower.

So many questions, too few answers

Yet despite the placebo effect's ability to trigger healing within us, as I studied more, nobody seemed to understand how or why it works. Nor had there been any real large scale research studies. I needed answers, so I decided to embark on a mission to learn more about the placebo effect and figure out what was really happening.

After years of intense practical and theoretical research, starting at the very beginning of my career, I'm proud to say I've found some of the answers and some very important questions that require further research. What I've discovered has been a revelation, and the inspiration for this book.

To be clear, I don't have all the answers. There is much more work to do and one of the motives behind this book is to encourage more high-quality research into this area.

But as soon as I realised the incredible potential hidden inside the placebo effect, I knew I needed to share what I'd learned. I applied this to my practice, started various projects that aimed to deliver this vital education, and worked tirelessly to get the word out and help people to empower themselves. After two decades, I would like to suggest a succinct and concise way that you may be able harness this superpower for yourself.

In short, the placebo effect is a testament to the power and the ability for the body to heal itself, and I have a growing belief that it is possible to access this power without the need for a clinical setting, for doctors' visits, overmedication, or placebo sugar pills. We can harness this superpower, in a meaningful and honest manner, ourselves.

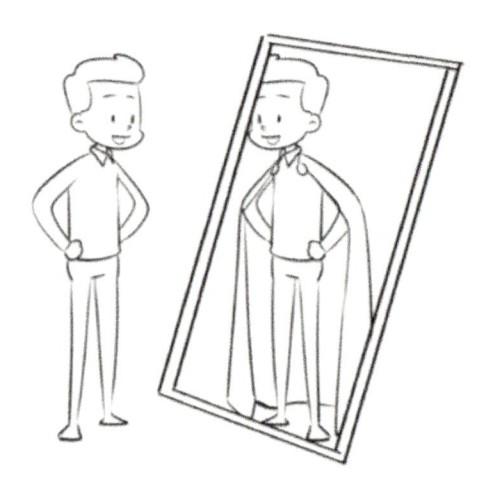

One of the interesting things that I realised early on in my research was that at the heart of the placebo effect was a shift in mindset. An *unhealthy* one transformed into a *healthy* one.

How easily this switch can occur is dependent on many factors. Your education, your belief system, your past conditioning, and your nature are all very important factors, as we can see from the literature in this area.

But there is one thing we are sure of...
The placebo effect is about the unconscious internal processing that occurs during a therapeutic intervention. I want to know how to harness this power, consciously.

The first and most important factor I found was, that the relaxation response was an important part of this process, a deep focused relaxation acts

30

as a reset for the mind and body. This reset can happen in many unconscious ways during a consultation but consciously the relaxation response was a powerful tool.

No matter how serious the condition is that we are suffering with, the ability to relax and let the body leave the fight-or-flight mindset is incredibly beneficial. The Relaxation Response has been studied extensively at Harvard University as far back as the 60s by Dr Herbert Benson.

Another important factor that I saw time and time again was a change in the level of a patient's 'Activation'. This usually involved a change in a person's mindset. Activated patients are more engaged, aware and proactive in their own healthcare and less of a burden to the NHS.

In many medicine/wellbeing systems around the world, a great deal of attention is paid to the life force. A strong life force equates to a healthy individual and a low life force leaves a person prone to, open to, or susceptible towards one illness or another.

The Life Force is central to many traditions. In Homoeopathy, Samuel Hanhemann termed it The Vital Force, in Hinduism and Ayurvedic medicine it is called Prana, in Buddhism and Chinese Medicine it is called Chi or Qi. A change in mindset can free up this life force and help to improve a person's health, energy and even happiness. Patient

Activation Measures are increasingly becoming an important and vital part of how the NHS hopes to work in the future.

And this leads nicely to the final aspect of the placebo effect and long-term behavioural change:

Self-care or Self-Management.

How can you maintain this change? The reset, the activation and the mindset change? This is when you fully step back and reflect about your life, and ask yourself:

'How can getting healthy help me get to my life goals?'

'What impact would a healthier, happier, stronger me, have on my life and my work?'

'How can I develop the mindset and behaviour that improves the chances of me, living a healthy, happy and fulfilling life?'

These are important questions. Vital questions. Questions that many of us haven't given necessary attention to answering. Now, what is the benefit of making the lifestyle changes in your life? Making a change can be difficult, extremely challenging and can upset the family setup and routines, i.e., making dietary changes for a type two diabetic parent, does the parent cook separately or make unpopular changes dietary for the whole family? Or how to find the time to exercise in an already busy schedule etc. Why would you make such an effort? What is the point of giving up on my few pleasures in life? Is there any motivation for the change? It's a question few of us ever consider.

Returning to the doctor's consultation, that moment when you get the diagnosis, you might realise how much your health really means to you. ==You realise all kinds of goals you have to live a better life, to earn more money so you are no longer just surviving but thriving in life.== Maybe your goal is to see your grandchildren grow up, or to stay mobile in old age, or maybe you have some life mission or purpose that you must achieve.

As we move through this book, I'll show you how you can make the placebo effect work for you using my proposed model. Crucially, I'll show you just how much the placebo effect can bring to your life and how to use it starting today.

The placebo effect is proof that it's possible to put the mind and body back on track, to bring them both into alignment with your goals, and harness your innate superpower to improve the quality of your life.

This book will educate you about how it can be done and increase your odds of living a full and healthy.

33

Chapter One:
Your Body Is an Incredible Piece of Kit

"If we did all the things we are capable of we would literally astound ourselves."
— *Thomas Edison*

By the time he was three years old, Jordan Harden had spent most of his life battling leukaemia. Doctors gave him only weeks left to live. It looked certain that his life would be cut short when it had barely even begun. Every new piece of news had become too much to bear. Jordan's family told the hospital to stop calling with test scan results, giving themselves some space to take a break from the stress and upset. Instead, knowing their little boy's time was running out, the family opted to take Jordan to Disneyland Paris for a final family holiday.

Then, just days before they were set to leave for the holiday, Jordan's family got a phone call with some astonishing news: His cancer had gone.

The scans were clear and all indicators negative. What happened to Jordan is known as spontaneous remission, where people recover from cancers and other diseases with either no treatment or a treatment that couldn't cure the patient on its own.

35

While relatively rare, there have been other cases of spontaneous remission in many kinds of cancers, as well as other seemingly incurable diseases, like HIV and arthritis. One organisation, the Institute of Noetic Sciences, has collected records of more than 3,500 cases of spontaneous remission reported in the medical literature over decades. Each of these fascinating cases are proof of the human body's ability to overcome seemingly insurmountable odds.

Beating cancer in time for a Disneyland trip seems like it should be impossible, but Jordan's case, like many of the other spontaneous remission cases documented so far, is proof that it can and does happen.

It is my belief that the power that led to Jordan's recovery, and to so many other spontaneous remission cases, lives in all of us. I also believe it's the same power that drives the placebo effect. And once we can harness that power, we can use it to bring health and healing into our daily lives.

It is important to point out that what we are looking at here is not a one size fits all, nor am I saying everyone can be cured. The point is to recognise that we can increase the odds in our favour, we can prepare ourselves to heal, and maybe, just maybe it may trigger the body to do something spectacular. The mind is very complex. And changing one's mind is even more complex.

We don't know what exactly went on inside the heart and mind of Jordan Harden. Was it the acceptance of the prognosis? Was it the excitement of the trip that 'activated' his lifeforce? We don't really know. Booking a trip to Disneyland for another child in a similar position probably won't have the same results. But the interesting thing that researchers have found is that children are more responsive to the placebo effect than adults.

Everyone, young and old, have different motivational threads, pressure points and learnings (education, family values, social media etc). This makes it virtually impossible to say a course of action that works for one person will necessarily work for another. In my opinion this is the biggest short coming of the Western Medical Model, one size doesn't fit all. Although, personalised patient centred care is the direction things are moving towards, this is very slowly and faces many challenges.

What is becoming increasingly clear is that it isn't as important which treatment, medicine or therapy is used as it is whether the patient ready and prepared to make the changes needed.

Imagine, we have a patient with Type 2 Diabetes. After a few months of medication, the condition is controlled but the patient continues to eat poorly, a diet that consists of too many sugary processed foods. What can the doctor or medicine do if the cause of the illness is never addressed?

Having said that, the food patients are given in hospital in this country is nothing short of criminal. In one instance, a young boy, who was hospitalised due to diabetes Type 1 complications, was given sugary cereal for breakfast. When the mother complained, the nurse apologised and gave him a banana instead. The lack of resources and education available is so poor, it's become a case of the blind leading the blind.

It is important to notice if any therapeutic intervention works to switch off the fight/flight system, activate the life force (by changing the mindset) and encourage a patient to make meaningful lifestyle choices. Once a patient has been prepared in this way, we can see effortlessly how any further therapy (pharmacological or otherwise) would yield even better results.

Without doubt, the most important factor is how we process events in our mind. Despite the challenges we may face at any time, can we unlock our minds to realise our potential and increase the odds in our favour? Can we create the space, the time, and the opportunity for our body to heal?

As Emile Choe, the prominent French pharmacist and psychologist, put it:

'It is more important what you say to a patient than what you give to a patient'.

My experience says this is true. When my interventions leave the patient feeling relaxed, reassured, activated, and prepared to heal, the chances of positive health outcomes increase quite dramatically.

I am certain that as you read through this book you will also find strong evidence to support this statement. When our mind and our body are aligned to heal us, the results are nothing short of miraculous. Jordan's story, along with thousands of other cases, are proof such miracles are possible.

Unfortunately, an unhealthy mind or a negative therapeutic intervention can turn that same power against us. If we consider that the placebo effect is considered a desirable outcome then we must consider the opposite also, the nocebo effect, placebo's evil twin. The nocebo effect is also a recognised phenomenon, with opposite results to the placebo effect, where a therapeutic intervention causes poor health outcomes.

The mind is not separate from the body, as we sometimes imagine it to be. Instead, the health of one directly influences the health of the other. Pessimism, fear, and stress all contribute to internal pressures that directly and indirectly affect a person's sense of wellbeing, as we have already seen with the fight/flight response. When the mind is healthy, the body tends to be healthier as well. In the same way, improvements in physical health often improve mental health as well.

A good example of this is how people with depression can improve their mental health through exercise.

The conventional thinking is that depression is caused by low levels of Serotonin. But researchers have found that exercise causes the body to produce more Serotonin, alongside other mood-boosting chemicals, which help to increase feelings of happiness.

In fact, studies indicate that exercising three times per week to the point of perspiration (a proper good work out) may be more effective than antidepressants when it comes to the effect on Serotonin levels and hence exercise is better at improving the mood and wellbeing of a person than drugs.

After all, antidepressants such as Fluoxetine (sold under the brand name Prozac) and Sertraline (aka Lustral) can only stop your body reabsorbing and breaking down the Serotonin it has already made. Exercise also avoids some of the nasty side-effects of antidepressants. There is a very interesting choice here. Is the best strategy to try and stop the body breaking down old Serotonin or would we prefer to encourage our body to make more?

I am not, of course, suggesting that we should avoid taking medication – the stigma around mental health is already so much of a burden. I know that when you're stuck in bed all day and, in some cases, barely able to summon the strength and will to leave the house, being told that you should try going for a run three times a week probably seems like a cruel joke. But doctors can move quickly to medication without mentioning the benefits of exercise at all.

Everyone deserves to know all the options open to them so they can choose which fits their personal goals and aspirations, as well as the reality of their situation. Only then can we move to a health system which is patient centric and based on informed choice. Shared Decision Making and Patient Centred Care are already high on the NHS's agenda for change.

Can you invoke healing superpowers at will?
Well, yes. The goal with this book is to explore how you can do this by harnessing the placebo effect, consciously. In doing so, you'll be learning a skill that will benefit many areas of your life in the future. Many people have been doing this all their life, unconsciously. Now, we can learn to do it consciously. Here's a very simple example:

Let's imagine you are in your kitchen, chopping onions with a knife, when there's a sudden knock at the door. The knife slips in your hand, slicing into your finger and leaving a cut.

Straight away, your body responds to the injury, rushing to protect you. Blood wells up out of the wound, and special blood cells called platelets begin to link up and clot together, drying out to create a scab. This quickly stops blood getting out and bacteria getting in.

Once the clot forms, your blood vessels then open so that oxygen rich blood can flow to the area and promote healing. Meanwhile, white blood cells known as macrophages head to the injury to gobble up any harmful bacteria that might have entered the body through the cut. These macrophages also make chemicals that help in healing.

More blood cells move to the wound and help you to grow new tissue, while our bodies make a protein called collagen. Collagen then acts as a scaffold for other tissue to grow around. Eventually, the tissue gets stronger until all signs of the cut have vanished.

It happens all the time, and yet it is an incredible feat. Think of the millions of years it took for such a complex system to evolve, coming together to create this astonishing ability.

Left to its own devices, the human body is a natural healing machine. It knows what to do. It's something we all know, but rarely think about. As we move through the world, we don't worry about cuts or scrapes. Even more serious injuries like a broken leg can heal in just six to eight weeks. The capacity to repair ourselves lurks in all of us and isn't just limited to injuries.

In fact, our bodies even fight off potentially cancerous cells all the time. Since cancer is caused by mutations in the DNA inside our cells, we've evolved ways to detect these mutations and repair them. Our immune systems are also experts at finding and destroying potentially cancerous cells before they can cause problems.

We have other cancer-fighting abilities as well. Since the sun's rays damage DNA, and can cause mutations, skin cells that detect this damage will essentially self-destruct, so they don't turn cancerous.

When something in our body's systems goes wrong, or gets overloaded, that's when problems emerge. It's unfortunate that, instead of reflecting on what we are capable of, we only really experience the body through these problems. When everything is working as it should, we don't think of our bodies at all. We take ourselves and our bodies for granted. It's only sickness and pain that catches our attention and pressures us to act.

Our bodies are wonders, and if we can learn to live in harmony, we would experience many joys and benefits that are the result of living a healthy life. Every day they heal and sustain us. And it's a thankless job, since we rarely acknowledge the everyday miracles that let us live in a world full of sharp edges, deadly infections, and many other hazards to our life.

What's more, there are plenty of industries willing to support us in viewing our bodies as faulty or damaged. Medical care in the UK has become much the same. Our only exposure to healthcare comes when we're sick, with little to no effort or investment in keeping us healthy.

People within the health system often joke amongst themselves – the NHS isn't the National Health Service but the National Treatment Service. Isn't it fascinating that even after years of education and training, experts are fully versed in disease progression but not so much in the development of health or the prevention of ill health?

Of course, for all the body's self-healing powers, we still get sick. It is still possible to get a whole host of other illnesses. Clearly, things can and do go wrong. As we'll explore, though, it's not always the body that has gone awry when it comes to healing.

Often, it's the mind. It is estimated that up to 80% of long-term chronic conditions are psychosomatic. We have the origins of the problem within the mind (psycho) and body (soma), not just in the body alone. Errors in thinking can cause negative habits and behaviours. It is therefore clearly futile to focus any potential treatment on just the physical aspects of a disease without considering the deeper psychological aspects of a patient's condition.

==This mindset shift, from unconscious tension to a default relaxed state, is what triggers the healing effect.== This allows the body to realign itself, what's known as Homeostasis. If it is possible to correct one's thinking, surely this is the first step. The incredible thing about the relaxation response is that it gives the mind time and space to adjust and adapt.

When a threat hijacks the amygdala (the part of the brain that decision making and emotional responses) and kicks starts the fight/flight response a whole cascade of hormones and chemical changes take place (your adrenaline levels change, your blood pressure goes up, your breathing quickens, your insulin increases). Ultimately, the result is that your muscles tense up, which you can feel, and this tightness reflects to the mind, which, in turn gets tighter. Neural pathways create a negative cycle of anxiety, tension, and stress.

When the threat is no longer in front and the person hasn't reset the nervous system, this tension is unconsciously stored in the muscles and nervous system, over time more and more is stored and mind sets become fixed, the neural pathways repeat habitual thinking and actions based on flight/flight, often unhealthy behaviour, and at this point the chances of developing an illness increases.

Imagine when there are multiple stressors. The mind gets wrapped up in all these things. The energy (the *life force*) that would normally be involved in the normal functioning of the body is trapped elsewhere. Now, what if the mind relaxes, accepts the challenges being faced and frees up that energy. The mind and body get back into sync and the body starts to heal. The placebo effect happens subconsciously. But can we do this consciously.

Can we shift our mindset and get into sync with our bodies again?

Give me a break

We know that the body is always working to protect us from harm, healing injuries and fixing problems. However, the ways we live can make this much more challenging than it needs to be. Most crucially, our healing process gets interrupted by stress. Studies show that our bodies take longer to heal injuries when we're experiencing chronic stress.

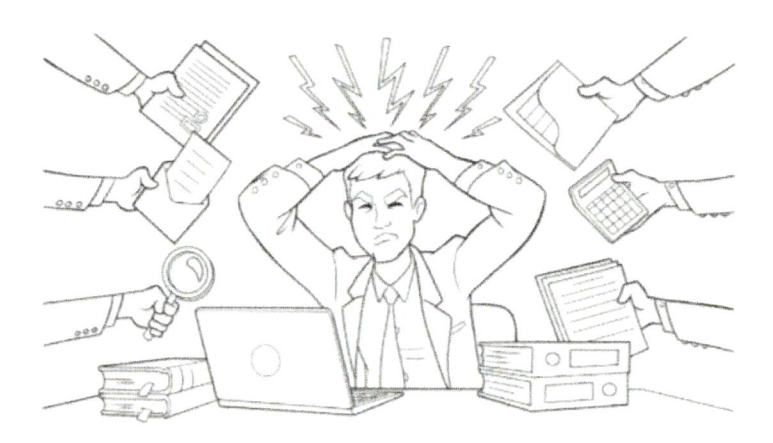

We have all experienced times when life events hijack our mind. But it is not just our minds and thinking that gets hijacked, but our very life force gets trapped in these repetitive patterns.

Without proper rest, it's impossible for us to recover. And rest doesn't just mean taking days off every now and again. And it certainly doesn't mean sitting in front of the TV, nor is it going outside for a cigarette or scrolling endlessly on social media.

I'm referring to something very specific: the relaxation response. As mentioned earlier, this was first described by Harvard physician Herbert Benson. The relaxation response is essentially the opposite of the fight/flight response.

While the fight/flight response ratchets up tension in the body, spiking blood pressure and flooding the body with stress hormones, the relaxation response does the reverse. It's a state of deep rest and calm, where the heart rate slows, blood pressure falls, muscles relax, and the body slips into the healing mode.

This response is a natural feature of the human mind which you can use to your advantage. There are multiple ways to enter this state of relaxation. In addition to transcendental meditation, there's also yoga, zen, and even hypnosis.

This relaxation response is one of the factors that connects all of these, many of which have existed in some form for thousands of years.

Benson studied people engaging in these and other similar practices and found changes in all sorts of areas of the body compared to those who don't. The important thing is that the relaxation can be learned. For some it will be easier than it is for others, but it is possible to be trained to relax.

Benson recommends inducing the relaxation response daily, opening the body up to healing and allowing us to leave our anxious mental and physical state behind. After all, without a way in day-to-day life to let go of stress, we're essentially putting the brakes on the body's stress response all the time – never giving ourselves the opportunity to use our innate healing ability at full power.

As we delve further into the placebo effect, and how to use it, keep relaxation in the forefront of your mind. It has a pivotal role in the process.

Think of yourself like a jug of water set on a table. The challenges of your life are like glasses you must fill, always in need of more water.
When you are careful to take time and refill, then you have water to spare – you can take on challenges with ease.

48

You can't pour from an empty jug

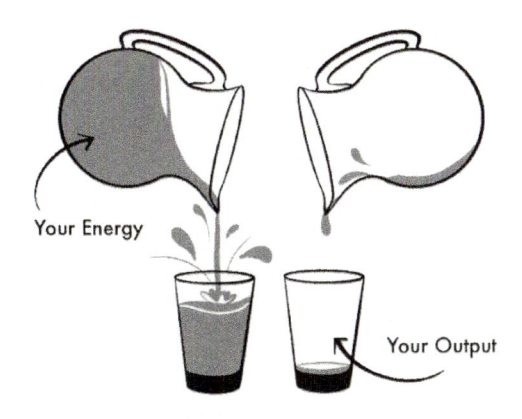

Your Energy

Your Output

We could make another analogy. At what point do you reach for the charger when your phone battery is low? If you don't take that time to replenish, to recharge, you can empty yourself out completely. Moreover, once the water is gone, the challenges of life become that much harder to handle – maybe even impossible.

As they say, a hungry man can't feed the world. We must make sure that we fill ourselves up with lifeforce and energy, and then develop daily practices to ensure the energy is always high.

Without rest and relaxation, you will always feel emptied out and exhausted. And at that point, you are far more susceptible to illness. I hope this book can offer more than one piece of advice. But if there was only one lesson here, this is it: rest is the foundation upon which the placebo effect is built.

Without quality deep relaxation, it is fundamentally impossible to achieve a healthy body or a healthy mind. Proper rest. Rest that can, over time, desensitise the fight/flight system, so it doesn't fire so easily.

There is also growing evidence that relaxation, rest and meditation can create an environment for Telomeres to lengthen and repair. Telomores are the caps at the end of your chromosomes, which protect your DNA. Going deep into this is beyond the scope of this book, but there is a lot of interesting research available on this too.

As we delve into the placebo effect even more, and how you can unlock its powers, remember that rest and your life force are paramount. Consider how your mindset and behaviours would be different when you prioritise these two vital important factors in your life.

Chapter Two:

What Is the Placebo Effect?

"The effectiveness of a placebo is directly related to the impression that it makes on the subconscious mind."
— Dr John Sarno

The history of the placebo effect goes back as far as humans have been alive, creating a multitude of unbelievable but true stories. Still, the tale of Mr Wright must be one of the most astonishing.

Mr Wright's story appeared in one of the most famous papers ever published, documented by Dr Bruno Klopfer in the *Journal of Projective Techniques*. If it hadn't been documented so extensively, with multiple medical scans, I doubt anyone would have believed it.

Wright had lymphosarcoma, a cancer of the lymph nodes. The cancer was advanced and had spread throughout his body, wreaking terrible damage. The man was filled with tumours as big as oranges, leaving him bedridden and barely able to breathe.

When Wright entered a California clinic in 1957, having exhausted virtually every known treatment, doctors gave him only days to live.

However, in a stroke of luck, it was at this same clinic that Wright first heard mention of a drug called Krebiozen. At the time, this drug was typically given to horses, but it was under investigation as a possible cancer treatment.

Mr Wright quickly became convinced that this drug held the chance of a cure and begged to be included in a drug trial. Though Mr Wright's miniscule life expectancy made him ineligible for the Krebiozen trial, Klopfer ignored the clinic's rejection and prescribed Wright the drug anyway.

Much to everyone's astonishment, the drug seemed to be working. Mr Wright made a rapid recovery. Klopfer explained that *"the tumours had melted like snowballs on a hot stove, and in only these few days, they were half their original size!"*

Unfortunately, months into his remission, things went wrong for Mr Wright. Though the drug seemed to have miraculous results, newspapers were reporting something completely different. According to news reports, Krebiozen didn't seem to work at all.

As quickly as they'd vanished, Mr Wright's tumours soon returned. Somehow, his belief that the treatment wouldn't work had made him sick again.

Seeing this, Klopfer opted for an unusual strategy. He dosed up his syringe and injected Wright again – this time telling him it was a double-strength version of Krebiozen.

However, instead of a drug of any kind, Klopfer injected Mr Wright with water. In other words, Klopfer had given Wright a placebo.

Miraculously, Mr Wright's health soon returned, and his tumours vanished once again. The placebo seemed to have cured him.

All was well until, two months later, the American Medical Association declared Krebiozen "worthless" as a cancer treatment. Mr Wright was dead within 48 hours.

Wright's story makes a case not just for the body's ability to heal itself, but for the mind's role in that healing.

But, for all the benefits of the mind's powers of wellness, Mr Wright's experience also makes plain the mind's ability to make us ill. His absolute conviction that it would work had incredible results. At the same time, when he lost that faith, his health quickly declined.

Making the case for the Placebo effect

I'll let you in on a secret: the power of your own mind is as good as or better than most of the drugs humans have ever tested. I can say this with confidence because only a tiny minority of medicines manage to beat the placebo effect in drug trials.

Think about that.

There are all these big pharmaceutical companies spending astronomical sums to carefully develop new products, testing them out in lab-grown cells and mice and seeing exciting results all along the way.

Then, after all that time, they finally get to the point of testing their shiny new drug on humans and... it turns out that the human body is incredible at healing itself.

To explain why, I've divided the process of harnessing 'the placebo effect', consciously, into three key elements.

1. The Relaxation Response

To understand how to harness the placebo effect, we need to start with the relaxation response. After all, it's almost an antidote to the damage the fight/flight stress response does to the body.

Often, we feel weighed down by our life problems, pushed into that fight/flight state. Our mind keeps going back to the problem, maybe even keeping us awake late into the night. But seeing someone empathetic and competent, someone who can reassure us that our health is safe in their hands, can finally end a potentially catastrophic stress response.

On top of that, medical care can trigger our bodies to at last enter the far more beneficial relaxation response. It's not just the end of stress that benefits us but this entry into a new state that is receptive to healing.

Based on my discoveries, and the voices of many experts in the field, it's clear that relaxation plays an enormous role in improving the quality of our lives and healing. In fact, when you truly realise the scale of the damage stress does to us, the importance of ending stress cycles begins to seem like the most urgent step towards a healthy life.

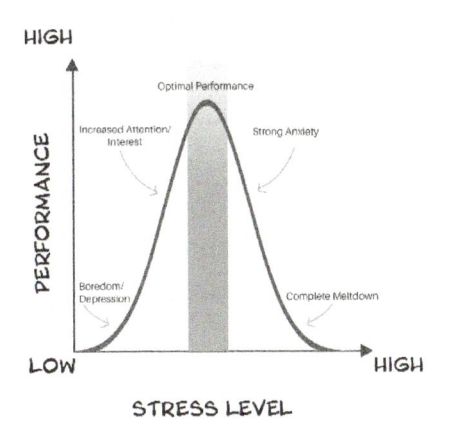

New research from the University of California, Berkeley, reveals an upside to experiencing moderate levels of stress. But it also reinforces how important it is to keep stress under control. The study, led by post-doctoral fellow Elizabeth Kirby, found that the onset of stress entices the brain into growing new cells responsible for improved memory. However, this effect is only seen when stress is intermittent. As soon as the stress continues beyond a few moments into a prolonged state, it suppresses the brain's ability to develop new cells.

Keep in mind that long term stress isn't just irritating, it's dangerous. Chronic states of stress can steal years from your lifespan and cuts down on precious days of good health. The impacts of stress span everything from headaches to more serious conditions like diabetes, all the way to strokes and heart attacks.

It is important to note here that some stress can be helpful in a person's development. It can add the right kind of pressure to give us a stimulus to act. The danger is when the stress becomes prolonged, overwhelming and/or not in line with a person's life journey.

The relaxation response is essentially a countermeasure against this damaging stress, bringing our bodies back into a state where they can heal and repair with far greater ease.

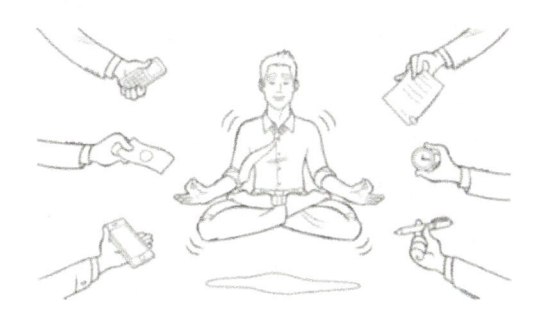

No wonder, then, that the reassurance of a kind doctor and a prescription for medicine – even when that comes in the form of a placebo – can be so beneficial.

However, I believe it's possible to go beyond what we've accomplished so far. Why should we need to see someone, or fill ourselves up with medicines, to access the placebo effect? The effect is born in the mind, not in the doctor's consultation room.

The relaxation effect dwells within us, it's not confined to the realm of medicine. Is it possible to train for relaxation? Yes, of course. Think of it like a muscle. If you don't use it, it shrinks, loses strength and power, but nothing a few heavy weight workouts won't change.

2. Activate your Life Force

The next key aspect, that I have witnessed, of harnessing the placebo effect is activating your Life Force. The stronger your Life Force, the healthier you are. We all have had those moments when something shifts in our thinking, and we find we are ready to make changes. Activation of the lifeforce covers not just energy levels, but also the skills, knowledge, self-belief, and desire to take responsibility for your health.

In the UK, people are in the doctor's consultation room for less than ten minutes on average. The rest of the time, everyone is pretty much on their own. The doctors effectively have one hand tied behind their backs. How on earth can we get down to the nitty gritty of life's messy parts, the things that might truly be making us sick, in under ten minutes?

I believe activation is another crucial aspect of harnessing the placebo effect. Whenever we see a doctor, it can be a major catalyst for getting us to engage with our own health and straighten out our thinking. In that moment, we realise that we have a choice: to continue as we are or to make changes for the better. What happens in the mind of a patient during a therapeutic encounter is at the heart of understanding the placebo effect.

For example, say a patient visits the doctor with nausea, headache, and light sensitivity. She diagnoses the patient with migraine.

Up until now, the patient had been getting by with over-the-counter painkillers and huddling away in their room. However, the diagnosis pushes them to re-evaluate the way they've been handling their migraines.

What if one of your friends then recommends a massage and you decide to give it go? You will experience the full sensory stimulus that comes with anticipation of a therapeutic benefit.

The professional massage setting, the smells of massage oils, the soft sounds being played in the background, the professional and caring demeanour of the therapist.

All this works together, with the actual massage process, to work away tensions that are being 'stored' in your muscles and, as you relax deeper, you have a sense of expanse as your mindset shifts and your thinking becomes clearer.

At the same time your body releases Serotonin, Oxytocin, Endorphins and Dopamine. You feel better. There is a cascade effect – psychosocial effects, actual therapy, hormone chemical release, which compound to switch your state and increase the odds of wellness in your favour. It allows you to relax even deeper.

This gives you to time and space to unravel. Your mind communicates within itself in a different manner. More holistically and ideas and insights start to pop into your head. The train of your thinking changes, from focusing on the problem to finding solutions. They find that inner strength and the 'will' to make some changes. The Life Force gets activated.

As Hippocrates said:

"The natural healing force within each of us is the greatest force in getting well."

As soon as you get home, you start reading up on migraines to improve your knowledge and understanding of the condition. It turns out that there can be all kinds of triggers for these attacks, ranging from diet, to sleep, to different medications.

You have started to learn what you need to do to stay healthy. You start to believe in yourself and the steps you can take to improve and manage your own condition.

Eventually you set about finding what's causing the migraines. Maybe you make changes to your diet with more migraine-friendly foods (reluctantly cutting out salty foods and aged cheese), as well as less alcohol.

With each change you make that reduces your migraines, you become more secure and conditioned to managing your health. When people offer you a food you've not had before, you are confident enough to ask the ingredients before eating to make sure they're migraine safe. It becomes your 'new normal.'

Thanks to your own research, and growing understanding of the condition, you manage to reduce migraine attacks from more than five times a month to just one. You have become an empowered, educated and an active participant in your own care.

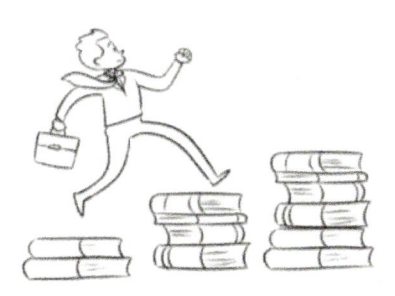

As you know we don't need to depend on doctors or placebos to become active in our own health. We can be active whenever we choose. When we are activated in the right manner there is an inner strength, a thirst to learn and to act. Eventually this becomes intuitive and more aligned with our inner voice, our inner knowingness. We become the masters of our own destinies.

3. Taking action

The final element of the placebo effect, to my mind, is self-care. This comes from asking the tough question: *Why bother?*

In a strange way, it can almost feel like a betrayal to decide to focus on our health. The way we live our lives comes from experiences, from family and friends, from our job and our education. It can feel like we're turning our back on those things if we suddenly change course.

We exist as we do for a multitude of reasons. If we're not exercising, or eating enough vegetables, or getting enough sleep, there are reasons for it. These patterns don't come out of nowhere, and their roots reach down into our sense of self. I think you would agree most people know what a good healthy lifestyle looks like, regular exercise, good nutrition, cut out toxic habits and foods, have a good social circle, have a purposeful and meaningful life. But how do we go about making those changes?

Ray Dalio, the co-founder of the world's largest hedge fund says that it is important to recognise that
 1) the biggest threat to making a good decision is harmful emotions and
 2) decision making is a two-step process, learning and *then* deciding.

To make changes that last, we must claw our way out of a lifetime's worth of habits and opinions.

To make things harder, just because we're making positive changes, that doesn't mean there are no downsides. Being the only one at work not going out for drinks on a Friday night can be a huge blow to someone's social life, or even hurt their chances of promotion.

Consider what Krishnamurti said:

"It is no measure of health to be well adjusted to a profoundly sick society."

For that reason, it's not enough to do things out of obligation. Ultimately, that way of thinking eventually takes us back the way we came – back to our old obligations, our old mistakes.

If we're going to manage this herculean task of changing, we must really want to change. I don't mean wanting some vague outcome of being 'healthier' but wanting more from life. We're not going to make a change if we don't, deep down, think it's worth it.

We need to believe, fundamentally, that health is one of our most important goals. And, more than that, that it has a central place in all our other aspirations. Managing our health – whether we are dealing with long-term health issues or not – needs to be a part of the life we imagine for ourselves.

That's not to say that disability, or injury, won't happen. All of us are mortal, and accidents happen. But we have the best chances of coping with challenges, of adjusting to the new shape of life, if we have worked to cultivate a healthy lifestyle.

Subconsciously, we often imagine ourselves in the future just as we are now. We don't account for how our habits in the present might come to impact our lives. Our plans to travel to a certain country; kick a football around with our children; have meaningful relationships; and perform well at work all depend on our health.

63

A doctor's visit can force us to reckon with that. It's why I consider it the third component of harnessing the placebo effect, consciously. However, there's nothing that says we need to wait for this reckoning until it's already started to affect our health. As Stephen Hawkings put it:

Intelligence is the ability to adapt to change.

When there are changes needed in your life, how easily are you able to adapt? Or do you resist the change and cause more internal stress?

Something can't be nothing

One other fundamental thing to understand about the placebo effect is that it's part of every treatment in medicine. It's part of how our minds work. But up until now, it's been an unconscious process.

In fact, I can guarantee you've experienced the placebo effect first-hand. Let's say, for example, that you have a headache. The pain is bad, so you decide to take a painkiller. While the drug takes at least fifteen minutes to start working, you find that you immediately begin to feel better.

Most of us can get our heads around the fact that that immediate feeling of relief when you first take the medicine is the placebo effect, but it's more than that. The truth is, even when the painkiller begins to work, the placebo is working underneath it.

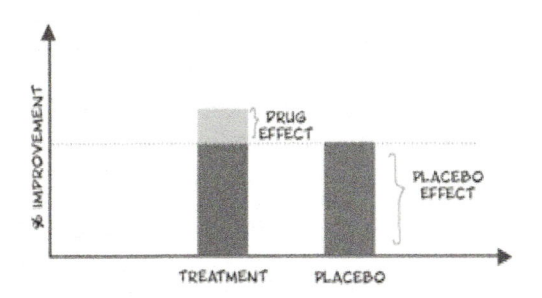

Adapted from Alia Crum's Tedx Talk

Why do we assume the placebo effect ends once the 'real' medicine kicks in? It makes no sense. The fact is that the total benefit of any drug is medication *plus* the placebo effect. With every medicine you've ever taken, you were essentially harness the placebo effect as well.

Bendetti et al (1995) also showed that the pharmalogical effect of a drug is greatly reduced when the psychological element is eliminated. Expectations are important.

Sensory stimuli have an important part to play in the placebo effect. It conditions the patient to 'expect' a therapeutic intervention to occur.

For example:

- **Sight:** seeing the doctor in a professional environment develops trust and confidence
- **Smell:** the distinctive smell of the surgery, hospital or clinic heightens the sense of being in the right place for treatment.
- **Words:** positive verbal suggestions cause the same neural pathways to be activated as when taking a powerful painkiller, for example.
- **Touch:** a good bedside manner as opposite to being cold and standoffish heightens the response.

Different social stimuli interact with the same neuro receptors as you would expect from taking a pharmaceutical agent.

If we look at the data from clinical trials and consider the improvements in a person's health, even when not taking a 'real' medicine, if it isn't the placebo effect responsible for the impact then what is it?

No wonder Dr Michael Dixon, chair of the College of Medicine, called the placebo effect "the most comprehensive, powerful effect that we have in medicine" when I spoke to him for this book.

Dixon believes that the placebo effect is a huge part of 'everyday practice' in the medical field but is unfortunately underestimated and under-researched.

==That would explain why we're only recently finding evidence for a mind-blowing aspect of the placebo effect: that placebos appear to work even when we *know* we've been given a placebo.== In fact, Dr Ted Kaptchuk, who researches placebos at Harvard Medical School, has studied so-called open-label placebos. That's where a patient is given a placebo and told that's what they're taking. His findings have already shown benefits to these open-label placebos in irritable bowel syndrome and lower back pain.

What this means is that the placebo effect isn't a trick. It isn't 'fake' medicine. There is something deeper going on. I am proposing that the therapeutic intervention causes a shift in the mindset of the person. This, I believe, is what causes us to witness the remarkable results that were witnessed.

The placebo effect has proven benefits that we've been ignoring for too long. Drug makers have been trialling placebos again and again against the medicines they've developed, and each time the placebo does better, they're disappointed.

But for us, it's the opposite of a disappointment. It means that, just like Mr Wright, we can see incredible benefits without needing any drugs at all. Ultimately, the placebo effect comes from within. It may seem like it must have an outside force to work, that you need a person with a lab coat and a bottle of sugar pills to gain access to its benefits, but really this ability has been inside you all along. The interaction between cognition and emotion are vitally important to achieving clinical therapeutic benefit, with or without adding any additional therapy to the therapeutic encounter.

What's more, I believe you don't even need to see a doctor to reap the benefits. Once you understand how the placebo effect works on your body, you can do it yourself without having to go out and buy a bunch of sugar pills.

Chapter Three:
How The Placebo Effect Became So Misunderstood

"In human intercourse the tragedy begins, not when there is misunderstanding about words, but when silence is not understood."
- Henry David Thoreau

Dr Alia Crum is the principal investigator at Stanford University's Mind and Body Lab. She's also one of the first people I came across who really began to reflect what I'd lived through when it came to the placebo effect.

She and her colleagues at Stanford have investigated how the placebo effect works across our whole body, changing all the fundamental processes going on inside us. The placebo effect acts on our hormones, our immune system, our breathing, and our digestion.

Not only that, but she's become just as fascinated as I have with the idea of intentionally heightening the placebo effect.

Crum was one of the first people I saw who really highlighted the ignorance of our current approach to the placebo effect in medicine. When humans discovered this power, we should have jumped for joy. Here's this incredible ability, this marvellous superpower lurking in everyone.

We should have been racing to unlock this potential at every turn, to bring it to the forefront of medicine. Instead, what did we do? We hated it.

We made the mark of a 'good' drug the ability to beat the placebo effect. As if, as Crum herself has pointed out, the placebo effect somehow stops working as soon as the 'real' effects of a drug kick in. Instead, she encourages us to view the placebo effect as the foundation that underpins the work of medications.

For example, Crum and her fellow researchers have found that when patients can see a nurse injecting a painkiller, they report much less pain than patients unknowingly dosed with the same amount by a machine.

This superpower, *Our Superpower*, can't just be written off as if it were nothing, as the establishment has done for many years. In her talks and interviews, Crum has pointed out the irony that we have decades of research on placebos, and yet until recently we had no idea how they worked.

Along with her fellow researchers, she has been working to unlock an explanation. Crucially, they've found that the benefits are only seen when the healthcare providers patients interact with are competent and warm. If doctors are fumbling, or appear incompetent, lacking in confidence or empathy, the effect can vanish.

70

Perhaps this goes some way to explaining why drugs often become less effective once they make it out of the trial stage and into communities. Life is chaotic. There's no way to guarantee we'll always have a good experience with an empathetic and experienced doctor. As a result, many of us leave our doctors' appointments unprepared to heal. And I think it's because we're failing to harness the power of the placebo effect.

If the placebo effect is what underpins medicine, then a poor experience leaves us with no foundation to build on. I believe this explains a mysterious phenomenon in modern medicine: somehow, we are managing to both overprescribe and under-medicate.

Patients frequently return to the doctor to say that a particular medication isn't working, and the doctor responds by adding a new one rather than taking any away. Over time, patients start to take a ballooning number of drugs, with fifteen percent of people in England taking at least five medicines per day. We're at the point now where doctors are prescribing new medicines to treat the side effects from other medications.

In 2021, an NHS England review found that one in ten drugs handed out by GPs and pharmacists offer no benefit to the patient whatsoever.

Over-prescribing can be dangerous. The more pills we're taking, the harder it becomes to spot harmful interactions, not to mention the increased chance of side effects. Perhaps two of them are safe to take together, but not if someone is taking a third as well. When you try to account for five or more medications at a time, it gets complicated quickly.

But I also said we were under-medicating. How can that be? Well, it's because half the medications prescribed aren't taken as directed. People skip doses or stop taking them entirely. In many cases, patients do this willingly. Non-compliance is a huge problem.

What I believe is happening, based on my own research and reading, is this: the drugs aren't working as well as they should, because, as Alia suggests, in real life they lose the structure and foundation for them to work.

Or maybe it is that the patient doesn't trust the doctor's recommendations, hasn't been adequately prepared to heal, or have the necessary structure for change (the placebo effect).

This is complex and we don't fully know all the reasons for a patient's non-compliance. But one thing is for sure, the psychosocial element is not working for the therapy to work.

Let's imagine there's a pharmaceutical company and they've just developed a brand-new drug. They take it through all the safety procedures, all the different trials, spending billions on development. The drug is working well.

The general rule of thumb for a placebo is that it's about 30% effective. So, for roughly one in three people, there's a benefit there even with a sugar pill alone. Great news for the pharma company, their drug is 10% better than placebo. It's a spectacular result, practically off the charts, the best the drug company could have hoped for.

Let's look at the maths there for a second though. If the sugar pill is 30% effective, and the new drug is 10% more effective than placebo, then that makes the actual medication 40% effective, right? Not quite so high after all. Unfortunately, that isn't how these drugs are working in real life scenarios.

In the clinical trial all the participants were taking the medicine like they were supposed to. In the real world, as we know, only half the patients who get prescribed the new medicine take it as intended. So, when you calculate the effectiveness of the drug as it's taken in the community, it falls to half of what it was in the trial: 20%. Which, as you can see, is in fact less than the 30% effectiveness of the placebo alone. I accept that this is a rather crude calculation, and I am only using to make a point. And the point is valid.

That means the NHS is spending billions per year on a system that doesn't work in real life as it does in the lab. There are obvious reasons, such as no financial reward for a patient in the community setting like there is for a clinical trial participant. Nor is there any excitement that a clinical trial patient may have about being 'picked' and 'paid' to try a brand-new ground-breaking treatment.

We must train our doctors to understand the importance of harnessing the placebo effect in every therapeutic encounter and to approach their patients in a totally different manner. A manner that can help build a foundation for healing. Dr Michael Dixon calls this the 'Human Effect.'

The smart people at Stanford, like Crum, are focused on helping doctors and nurses to consciously make use of the placebo effect in healthcare. It's a noble goal, and an excellent target for researchers. However, my big ambition is for everyone to harness this healing superpower for themselves.

Often, we find ourselves at the mercy of factors beyond our control. These can be big things, like the whims of pharmaceutical companies or the changing winds of politics, or something as seemingly small as whether our GP ate lunch that day or is a crisis of their own. We can't control these things. We can't sit back and just hope that the doctors and nurses around us treat us well and give us the necessary support to make the changes.

What we can do is give ourselves our best chance by igniting our own life force, cultivating that brightness inside ourselves that wants to thrive. I am not for a second suggesting that illness is our fault, or that harnessing the placebo effect will heal all wounds or re-grow missing limbs. For me, thriving means that we are alive to the world, its possibilities, and our own potential. That includes our potential for healing, to the fullest extent we can.

Fundamentally, I think the problem is that the NHS has a poor view of what it means to be healthy, and perhaps an even worse view of what it means to be human. The NHS, as it stands today, sees 'health as the absence of illness.'

This may be partially due to the atheist scientific mindset that the medical model is based on. This mindset doesn't consider the spirit, the lifeforce, or the true impact of a patient's power. In modern medicine, everything is organic.

This, in my honest opinion, is a real problem when it comes to healing. You see, health isn't about sickness. It's about joy, vibrancy, energy, connection. Health is about our relationship to the world, to each other, and to ourselves.
Health is about thriving in life.
A better definition could be the World Health Organisation view that health is 'a state of complete physical, mental, and social well-being and not merely the absence of disease and infirmity.'

There's an old Indian saying that sums it up well:

"Every person is guaranteed to die, but there's no guarantee that every person will live."

Viewing health as an absence of illness is fundamentally flawed. It causes us to see health as a kind of featureless shadow, with none of the light and colour a healthy life should possess.

This flawed thinking can worsen the experience of elderly, disabled and chronically ill patients. If the system treats health as an absence of sickness, then there's no understanding of what health even means for someone whose illness will not go away.

The placebo effect isn't nothing…it's our SuperPower

In 2019, global spending on research and development of drugs totalled $198 billion, a jump of 45% from $137 billion in 2012. Unfortunately, most of this funding goes into imitating other drugs already on the market. Only 11% of new drugs approved by the FDA were truly innovative.

Many are simply copies of existing drugs. A single drug takes more than a decade to develop and around $1 billion to make. For all those expensive, time-consuming drugs, the gold standard is to beat the placebo in just two clinical trials.

Two.

At first, that seems kind of counter intuitive.

The thing to beat is…nothing at all? It doesn't sound like a fair fight. Here's a drug that's been ten years in the making, sometimes even engineered for a specific target we know is associated with an illness. It seems like the drug should obviously beat the placebo.

But that's not what happens. At the latest stages of a trial – when so much time and money has already been spent, half the drugs tested can't beat placebo. Even though I've spent so much of this book so far talking about how amazing the healing power of our bodies truly is, it still seems extraordinary on some level.

When I think of the amount of money and all the intelligent people with their PhDs pouring hours of time and experience into the pharmaceutical industry, I can't help but be astonished. All of that, and yet the placebo effect manages to be just as good, or even better, a lot of the time.

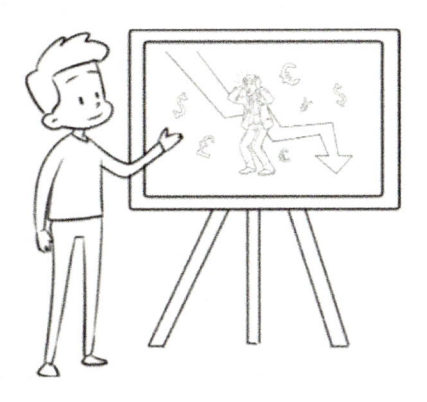

'I'm afraid that the drug failed to beat placebo'

It goes to show just how immense the power of the placebo effect is. Or, as I hope I've been showing so far, how important, and overlooked, the mind is when it comes to our health.

Despite this, we're often so dismissive of each other's attempts to bring the placebo effect into our own lives. We're reluctant to use this ability. I expect it's because everything we've heard about placebos in medicine makes them seem useless.

Let's say, for example, you've heard peppermint tea is good for digestion. Next time you get a stomach-ache you decide to give it a try. As you drink the tea, there's a pleasant tingling sensation in your mouth and throat from the mint. You notice the contrast between the cooling feel of the mint and the heat of the tea itself.

Drinking the tea feels almost like meditation, as the strong smell and taste hold your focus. It gives you a sensory stimulus which can cause you to 'expect' something positive to occur.

You feel much more powerful knowing you're doing something therapeutic for yourself. Your stomach was hurting, but now you're taking action to fix it. Not only that, but drinking the tea helps you feel relaxed and grounded. It's no surprise, then, that you feel better straight away. Indeed, if there is a therapeutic effect of the peppermint tea, this will help to compound this feeling of wellness.

Wanting to share the good news, you later mention your miraculous cure to a friend. However, instead of thanking you for your helpful advice, the friend just rolls their eyes and says *'Oh, it's just a placebo.'*

First, if it's 'just' the placebo, then why are all these companies spending their billions measuring against it?

Second, a negative attitude to the placebo effect completely fails to account for the fact that it works! Even if the peppermint has no bearing on digestion, drinking the tea can help to put us in a better frame of mind for healing. The properties of the tea aren't the only elements that are important. What matters is the effect that's evoked inside us. When we find things that help us engage with healing, especially when they cost very little, why not embrace them?

Next time you hear that something is *'Only the placebo effect,'* try to think about what that really means. Beware of charlatans, of course, but the peppermint tea is a perfect example of when it might make sense to embrace the placebo effect. Why not decide that it is working for you, and that's a good enough reason to keep drinking it?

We need to take a new approach, one that focuses on ourselves as the source of the placebo effect. Instead of saying something is only a placebo, it might be better to say something like *'This helps me to heal myself,'* or *'This prepares me for healing.'*

79

We should put ourselves in the driving seat when it comes to our health.

We need a new definition
Typical definitions of the placebo effect make two key mistakes. The first is that they typically imagine that it only works when someone interacts with a placebo in some way – whether that's a sham surgery (cutting someone open and then stitching them back up without doing the procedure) or common sugar pills.

As Alia Crum has pointed out, the placebo effect is also active when we take other medications as well. Even those with robust evidence. Every day, effective drugs like paracetamol and ibuprofen make just as much use of the placebo effect as fake treatments.

The second mistake in common definitions is the way they frame the placebo effect as something that happens to us, rather than something that comes from within us. I think this framing leaves little scope for imagining how we might understand and harness the placebo effect to improve our lives.

With these flaws in mind, I'd like to offer a new definition, a definition that needs thorough research to explore how we can harness this power in a meaningful manner to improve the quality of life in a patient:

80

A possible new definition for The Placebo Effect

This Placebo Effect creates a psychological reset causing a mindset shift, a change in consciousness, that allows the body to achieve a state of homoeostasis which can cause an improvement in a patient's condition.

When it comes to a new definition of the placebo effect, we're also left wondering why it works. As Crum has pointed out, the placebo effect doesn't happen at random. Instead, it appears to be what prepares us to heal – the scaffolding that medicine is built around.

Of course, we are all different, and what triggers the placebo effect in each of us varies from person to person. For that reason, it's been difficult to discover a clear mechanism of action for the placebo effect. After all, we each have different reasons to seek medical help, different levels of education, and different motivational threads underpinning our lives.

A one size fits all model of the placebo effect would be impossible. While we know that there are all sorts of factors involved in activating the placebo effect in each of us, there's not enough research to make any guarantees. Still, we do know what factors influence whether we'll hit all three placebo effect stages: rest, activation and self-care.

We know that communication between the doctor and patient is vital. When doctors are trustworthy, have a good bedside manner, show empathy, and listen to us, that puts us on the path to healing.

The placebo response could be triggered unconsciously, a conditioned stimulus, repetitive associations create the effect over time, or it could be conscious, where the patient has anticipation of therapeutic benefit.

Another important factor is our own expectations. Our fears, past experiences, and our beliefs about the world have a big influence on how well we can make it through the different placebo effect stages. Past traumas might make it harder for us to adapt to change, while a positive attitude to life might help us engage with healing. The wonderful thing is that it is possible to 'condition' yourself to 'expect' better results.

When we're aiming for a healthier life, it's important to keep individual psychology in mind. We must take culture, memory, emotions, and resilience into account. When we spot doctors, nurses, and other healthcare providers who are more skilled in navigating patients through each stage of the placebo effect, we need to take notice. We need to make a conscious effort to learn from these people and try to consciously replicate their success.

Chapter Four:
Health Is an Inside Job

"Every human being is the author of his health or disease."
— Swami Sivananda

Illness is often rooted in the mind. Studies have shown that 80% of long-term conditions (LTC) are psychosomatic – meaning they originate in the mind. The problem here is that people often take an unsympathetic view of these kinds of illnesses.

There are a whole host of reasons why this attitude is completely wrong. First, as we've discussed, illness is often the result of the wrong kind of stress. Whether that's a stress that results in high blood pressure, or stress that results in mental illness such as anxiety, or stress caused *inside* the body because of poor diet or a lack of exercise. The fact is every person who is sick deserves compassion and understanding.

Stress can literally shut down the body's ability to heal itself. It directly affects breathing, metabolism, insulin sensitivity, blood pressure, heart rate, and increases levels of stress hormones such as cortisol and adrenaline.

Second, just because an illness originates in the mind doesn't make it someone's fault. ==Major depression, for example, is a mental illness==. But given that it frequently drives people to self-harm and suicide, it's frankly disturbing to imagine that someone is bringing such suffering upon themselves.

Third, as time goes on, we're finding more and more links between the mind and body when it comes to health. It might even be somewhat reductive to make a clear separation between a mental illness and a physical illness. After all, as much as a third of people diagnosed with serious medical conditions also experience depression symptoms. In short, the chances of us getting from a LTC increases with poor lifestyle choices and errors in thinking.

All of this explains the growing respect for psychoneuroimmunology, also known as PNI, a science that focuses on how our psychology influences our bodies. The name is a bit of a mouthful, but when broken down into chunks it does a good job of explaining the basic idea.

Psychoneuroimmunology is the science of how the thoughts we have (that's the psych part) influences the nervous system and brain (hence neuro) and alters how the body fights disease (immunology). A key concept here is that our thoughts feed down through the mind into the body, while the body in turn sends signals back to the brain.

It has been shown numerous times that positive suggestions and other psychosocial factors, during a therapeutic intervention, can activate immune response, hormone release (GH, ACTH), endogenous opioids, and decrease stress hormones such as Cortisol.

PNI looks, among other things, at how outlook influences outcomes. For example, people with a more optimistic outlook tend to lead healthier lives (eating well, exercising, reduced smoking) compared to other groups, and are better at handling stress. They are more resilient to the changing fortunes in life.

Positive thoughts, then, lead to healthier habits and thus improve the chance of being healthy. Additionally, given what we know about the impacts of stress on the body, optimism would likely protect a person in other ways by reducing its impact on the body.

The more we learn about the mind-body connection, the more potential there seems to be in the placebo effect. After all, the placebo effect must be one of the best-known examples of the mind's influence on the body. It's the most obvious case we have where a person's thoughts result in better health. (Have a listen to Lissa Rankin's insightful TED talk *'Scientific Proof That the Mind Can Heal the Body.'* You'll find it fascinating.) Dr Dixon, Chair of the College of Medicine, said to me in conversation:

"We know that the physical can affect the mental, and so the placebo effect is in a great part our ability to use our minds to heal our bodies. We know that there are a vast number of ways of doing that – from the neuropeptides to the hormones, to the various whole pharmacology we have in our bodies of opiates and various things that almost mimic the pills and tablets that we give in commercial doses when we're treating people."

Our bodies have entire systems dedicated to reducing pain. Medicines like Morphine and Fentanyl only work because our bodies have an opioid system built in. We make our own opioids inside our bodies, called endogenous opioids, which help to relieve our pain.

What that means essentially is that within each of us, we can activate this system and modulate our own pain. In fact, that's what we are doing when we take a placebo, but we're told it's a painkiller. Science can prove it. If you give someone a drug called an opioid antagonist – a drug that blocks opioid receptors in the body – then the placebo won't work to stop pain. So, we know for sure that the body is activating our opioid system when we take a placebo.

And it's not just the opioid system that can be influenced by placebos. It goes way beyond that. So many medicines we take work on the systems we

86

already have inside us. I've already mentioned medications like Prozac, which work to stop the body from reabsorbing the serotonin it already made. You make the Serotonin, and you have the receptors for that Serotonin. Prozac just works with what you already have the power to make.

==The improvements we see from the placebo effect come from the biological processes that naturally occur in the body.== So, surely, there must be circumstances that trigger these systems to activate.

One of the most straightforward is known as conditioning. If you've ever heard of Pavlov's experiments on dogs, that was conditioning. He rang a bell each time the dogs were fed, and eventually just ringing the bell was enough to make the dogs start salivating.

Well, humans are not immune to being conditioned. We're conditioned to associate taking medicine with feeling better. If we take a placebo instead, our conditioning can still kick in. Our bodies then subconsciously activate healing processes in our bodies.

Dr Dixon gives the example of a patient whose sore throat always improves with an antibiotic like penicillin. Since most sore throats are caused by viruses, which aren't affected by antibiotics, it's very likely to be the placebo effect or a "self-limiting" condition, and not the drug itself:

"People know that when they take a foul-tasting tablet, and it's called penicillin, that makes them better. Therefore, by conditioned effect, they get better. So, it's a large number of different processes, which enable people to improve their immune system and increase their ability to self-heal."

But that's not the end of it. You see, we can condition ourselves. With time and patience, we can train our bodies to activate the systems that help keep us healthy.

That's why it's so vital to make the placebo effect part of our lives in an intentional way. Once you know that you can use your thoughts to improve your health, the next step is obvious. Although we can never say our health is entirely in our own hands, and for some of us the influence we have can seem very small, I believe we owe it to ourselves to take what power we do have and use it. For most of us, I think we have far more power than we realise.

The fascinating thing is that patients who are, traditionally, non-responders to the placebo effect can be conditioned, over time, to anticipate and expect benefits from a therapeutic intervention that can greatly increase the odds of them experiencing improved health outcomes.

88

When you get ill, you stop evolving.
In my time as an executive coach, one of the most helpful concepts I use with my clients is the idea of the flow state. The idea of the flow state was first presented by Mihaly Chikszentmihalyi.

He began to understand that people were their most creative, productive, and happy when they are in a state of flow. He interviewed athletes, musicians, and artists because he wanted to know when they experienced optimal performance levels.

Csikszentmihalyi developed the term 'flow state' because many of the people he interviewed described their optimal states of performance as instances when their work simply flowed out of them without much effort.

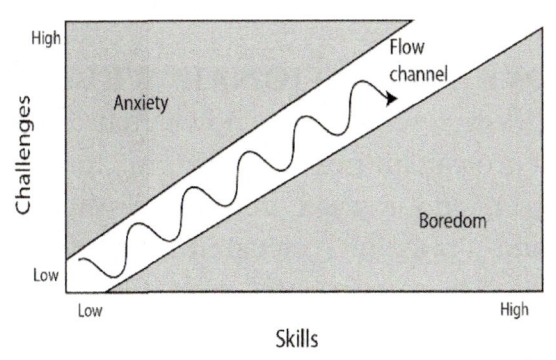

[Diagram: A graph with "Challenges" on the y-axis (Low to High) and "Skills" on the x-axis (Low to High). "Anxiety" is in the upper-left region, "Boredom" is in the lower-right region, and the "Flow channel" runs diagonally between them.]

Flow is a place, the sweet spot, the zone, where people can flourish in all areas. Remember the WHO definition of health being a state of optimal physical, mental, and spiritual wellbeing. Well, this is certainly pointing in the correct direction, wouldn't you agree?

If the challenges we face in life match up with our skill, then we remain in a flow state. If we aren't challenged enough to match our ability, then we become bored, stagnant, and lethargic. And if our skills don't match the challenge level then we become anxious, overworked, and overwhelmed.

Both are the opposite reactions and can cause internal stress: one is flight (not rising to challenges) the other is fight (addressing too many challenges).

In modern society both states are pretty much visible everywhere we look. The flow state is rare. But we see highly successful people live in the flow state and hear many athletes talking about being in the zone when they play their best. Maybe living in the flow state during life will bring out the best in you. When you are in the flow state, you are likely to experience:

IMPROVED EMOTIONAL WELL-BEING: State of flow research has shown that dopamine, a key neurotransmitter involved in pleasure, motivation, and reward, releases during the flow state and remains elevated afterward. This dopamine release correlates with a lasting sense of accomplishment and well-being.

HIGHER PRODUCTIVITY: Working in the flow state tends to be more efficient. When in a state of flow, you tend not to feel like you're trying at all and are less likely to get tired or bored. Also, the increased level of focus can make the task go faster.

GREATER LIFE SATISFACTION: People who regularly enter the flow state tend to have more life satisfaction. This could be a secondary effect from the positive experiences of flow, the satisfaction of achieving goals, or a combination of the two.

What has this to do with health you may ask. We all know that our bodies stop growing in our late teens. However, our minds don't. Nor should they. Life is always presenting us with challenges and impetuses for growth.

As we grow and learn we are better placed to overcome the challenges that we face and live a more fulfilling experience of life. However, what happens if we stop growing? The challenges will still be there, right? We must either run away from them or fight them.

Can you see how deep this goes? Not growing at the right pace, in the flow, causes stagnation. What is stagnating? You. Your very life force. And hence, your health.

One of the most common reasons I see for stagnation is when people are resisting growth. People may become overwhelmed with the challenges and become anxious. Or they shy away from the challenge and then the boredom starts to set in.

Perhaps a job that was once bringing us challenge and excitement has become unfulfilling, and we're resisting the change we need to make it right. Perhaps we need to push for promotion or embrace a new career entirely. It could be a personal challenge, too. Maybe we're reluctant to commit to a romantic partner or need to step up and help a sick loved one. Or maybe we need to get out of a toxic situation at work or at home.

In my experience, we all reach points where we become stuck. What's more, our stillness makes us ill. Our fears around the future, or apathy at the current situation, build up and keep us from flow. We become stuck, the stagnant energy around us keeps making us sicker. Our anxiety makes us more anxious, or else we become bored with our own boredom. It becomes a self-perpetuating cycle.

When we're unfulfilled, and unable to push for healthy change, we can end up turning to unhealthy ways to temporarily ease boredom or soothe anxiety. Perhaps we numb anxiety with alcohol or other drugs or spend hours scrolling through social media. If we've become bored, we might jeopardise our relationships with an affair.

When I meet people with these kinds of problems, it often matches up with the levels described in Maslow's hierarchy of needs.

SELF - ACTUALISATION
ESTEEM
LOVE
SAFETY
PHYSIOLOGICAL

You might have come across this idea before; it's typically explained using a pyramid with different levels.

It starts with our basic needs at the bottom, things like food and shelter, then moves up a higher level of living to feel safe and expressing yourself more authentically, then as we progress love and belonging becomes the most important goal, and so on up the pyramid.

A pattern I've noticed frequently is that when people need to move from one level to the next, that's when they're most likely to leave the flow state and veer off into boredom (flight) or anxiety (fight). They hit resistance. A subconscious glass ceiling.

In moments like these, we need to break through these mental blocks to progress to the next stage and keep on growing. Resisting the change is what causes all the problems. Refusing is what results in boredom or anxiety which then creates a cascade of events that increase the chances of a person getting ill.

When we are called to act, to adapt, we must do so. Anything else results in our bodies and minds not functioning as well as they could and could lead to illness in the long term. However, a simple mind set shift, a mental reset you might call it, can get us back into the flow.

In his book *The Biology of Belief*, Dr Bruce Lipton, a development biologist, talks about how changes in consciousness cause tangible measurable changes in the body.

I believe this is part of what happens during the placebo effect. That interaction with a nurse or doctor, in a sense, helps to unblock the way back to a flow state. It helps us accept that change is inevitable, and that we need to take the path ahead of us.

It is my sincere belief – coming from my experience in pharmacy and my time coaching – that flow is our natural state. Just take a look at children. They live in the flow state from one adventure and emotion to the next. They are constantly experimenting, growing and learning.

94

The question is, why do we get so precious with ourselves as we get older?

When we are in that flow state, accepting the challenges life has to offer us rather than trying to avoid them, we are healthier, happier, and more prone to achieving our goals. We are better at spotting the opportunities ahead of us, and better equipped to take them.

Time and again I find myself trying to help people go from where they are, to where they need to be, and it requires a certain kind of surrender to flow. Knowing that the most important thing is to be in the freshness of life, not squandering our time in stagnation or worrying our life away.

First, we must know where it that we want to go. What are our goals? We must develop a clear picture of what a healthy, happy, and fulfilling life would look like.

Of course, this takes time. We have been hurtling along life without to time to pause and reflect whether this path we are on is pointing in the direction that we want our life to go. We must stop and ask ourselves which way do we want to flow?

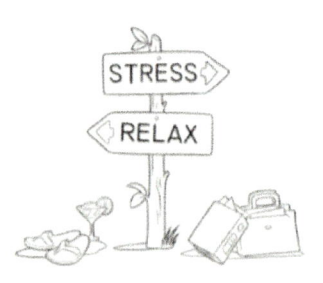

We must ask ourselves what would happen is we got off the hamster wheel of repetitive negative patterns and habits?

There's a common saying in psychology 'died at thirty, buried at sixty,' which pretty much describes the fate of people who can't make the changes needed for a fulfilling life. It's like Groundhog Day every day until death.

But health is about a vibrant life, it is about joy, it is about growth, it is about meaningful relationships with others and our work. However, we can't hope to achieve such a life when we refuse to accept change.

Looking at health, and the impact on the life of a patient in this context it is no wonder that Voltaire wrote over 300 years ago:

"Doctors pour drugs which they know little off, to cure diseases of which they know less into human beings of whom they know nothing."

This may seem harsh, but it gets the point across.

Despite the amazing achievements of the NHS over the past 70 years, the long-term conditions in the population are, worryingly, ever increasing. We'll tackle this thorny issue in the next chapter.

Chapter Five:
Pushback and politics

"The pharmaceutical industry isn't the only place where there's waste and inefficiency and profiteering. That happens in much of the rest of the health care industry."

- Marcia Angell

Elaine was the wife of a friend of mine and was diagnosed with motor neurone disease. They told her she had just six months to live, as the disease was progressing fast.

With motor neurone disease, muscles grow weak and stiff, eventually wasting away so that a person struggles to speak, move, eat, and even breathe. It is incurable and kills half of those diagnosed within just three years. However, some people will live much longer. Famous physicist Stephen Hawking, who lived to the age of 76 after a diagnosis at age 21, is probably the best-known exception.

My friend came to me after his wife's diagnosis and asked for my help. He told me the doctors had said there was nothing more they could do, so they were looking for other options. Even if there was no cure, it should still be possible to improve her quality of life and lift her mood.

I spoke with Elaine and, after a long consultation, the two of us came up with an action plan that included Tai Chi for movement, better nutrition, acupuncture, and regular guided relaxation classes. Thanks to our work together, Elaine's grip managed to strengthen, though not fully, and her walking improved. She was more stable on her feet, too. On top of that, her mood and her confidence improved, and she seemed much happier. Happier until her next check-up, anyway.

In our time together, she seemed to be doing well, but her visits to the hospital were another story. Elaine had to attend check-ups at the hospital every month, and each time she came back looking worse and worse. Her head would be down, shoulders hunched forward, and the spark in her would be dimmed to almost nothing.

Elaine's hospital visits clearly rattled her. She told me how she'd sit there, surrounded by other patients who were getting worse and worse, enduring pitying looks from the nurses. They saw her as a victim, which made her see herself as a victim too. She had to keep breaking free of that mindset again and again, each time more difficult than the last.

Fundamentally, I believe the doctors and nurses at the hospital were trying to help. They thought they were doing the right thing and trying to express sympathy for all the patients in their care.

For Elaine, though, it seemed the experience there did more harm than good. Nonetheless, Elaine far outpaced expectations. Given just six months to live, she survived eighteen months until a fall eventually sapped her of her energy, her confidence and belief.

What I learned wasn't just the importance of mindset when it comes to recovery, but also the attitude of the people around us. Without her husband and I working to build her up between visits and help her see the positives in her life, I think she could well have deteriorated much faster.

There are so many conflicting interests when it comes to healthcare, too many short appointments to discuss serious illnesses. When we only look at people as problems to be solved then an apparently "unsolvable" problem, like a terminal illness, becomes demoralising both to the doctor and the patient.

Since they can't be free of disease, and thus can't be healthy in the current view, we see any attempts to help as almost wasted effort. It's a strange attitude when you think of it.

All of us are mortal. Since we're all going to die anyway, isn't every treatment on the planet just postponing the inevitable? Why take a pitying attitude to Elaine just because she was closer than the rest of us?

The answer, I think, is that without a product to sell her, pharmaceutical companies aren't interested. She's not a customer anymore, making her worthless to these major corporations. Indeed, seeing how she was unconsciously treated made me incredibly sad. In many ways, this attitude has turned medicine into something cold and impersonal.

The problem with Big Pharma

If you wanted to use a single word to describe what's wrong with Big Pharma right now, that word would be 'money.'

I don't mean to say that most, or even many, of the people involved in the pharmaceutical industry are driven by greed. The people involved in pharmaceuticals are incredibly intelligent. Like doctors, these are very smart people who really could succeed in any industry. They could be raking in fortunes in banking, or law, but instead they've chosen to spend their days trying to find ways to improve the lives of their fellow human beings.

Unfortunately, when the desire to do good and the need to make money compete, money usually wins. There are plenty of ways for decent and well-meaning doctors and researchers to accept offers of food and funding, or to accept financial rewards for prescribing a medicine, and sincerely believe these "perks of the job" have no bearing on their decisions. After all, the world is not so neatly divided into 'good' and 'bad' people.

This business model is wrong. As Dr Aseem Malhotra, cardiologist and president of PHC so clearly said at the 2022 PHC conference: the business makes good people do bad things, often without them even realising.

In the UK many of the worst practices have been curbed in recent years but the power of Big Pharma in influencing the hearts and minds of people is stronger now more than ever. As we saw during the covid pandemic. $5bn was spent on lobbying in the US alone.

If more doctors are prescribing the drug, that's more money coming into the company that makes it. This extra money, in turn, gives the company the funds to influence more significant figures through lobbying and donations. Then, as more money funnels up the top, pharma companies start to offer high-paying jobs to former regulators. This creates an obvious incentive for regulators to approve drugs.

The problem doesn't stop there, either. It's Big Pharma that pays for most of the medical research. Most of the time, the company that makes the drug is the same company that tests it. This creates an inherently biased system for testing how safe and effective medicines are.

What's more, the scientists writing up their findings for medical journals are hugely incentivised to make their analysis as positive as possible.

Did you know that only about 43% of drug trial data is ever published? When submitting data for approval, a company is not compelled to provide all the information. Often unfavourable data is omitted.

What this means is that not only have doctors been highly incentivised to prescribe certain drugs, but most of the information available about these drugs comes from the pharma companies themselves. Within such a system, doctors' intentions start to matter less and less. They're surrounded by biased information. How can anyone make sound decisions based on incomplete data? Consider the words of Richard Horton, editor of *The Lancet*:

"*...possibly half of the published literature may simply be untrue.*" or this from Dr Marcia Angell,

"It is no longer possible to trust much of the clinical research that is published or to rely on the judgement of trusted physicians or authoritative medical guidelines. I take no pleasure in this conclusion, which I reached slowly and reluctantly over my two decades as an editor of The New England Journal of Medicine."

And this is when all parties play strictly by the rules and fines are already costed into the business model. When companies go further and push more aggressively, the potential for harm grows that much more.

GlaxoSmithKline (2012)
The charge: Illegal promotion of drugs.
The fine: $3 billion (largest fraud fine ever).

Pfizer (2009)
The charge: Off-label promotion "with the intent to defraud or mislead"
The fine: $2.3 billion (the largest fine of its kind).

Eli Lilly (2009)
The charge: Several lawsuits in various states resulted.
The fines: $1.4 billion, $25 million, and $22.5 million (reduced from $2 billion for violating use of a product label approved by the FDA).

Abbott (2012)
The charge: No scientific evidence existed to support their claims.
The fine: $1.5 billion.

Merck (2011):
The charge: Illegally promoted a treatment for rheumatoid arthritis despite any approval. The company also made misleading statements about Vioxx's effect on heart health.
The fine: $950 million.

It becomes much easier to hide dangers of certain drugs, including potentially fatal side effects, when companies have complete control over the narrative.

There's also much less chance of getting caught for misreporting findings, of making exaggerated claims.

Ultimately, the power of market forces in Big Pharma has gone unchecked for so long it seems impossible to control. While these companies do produce lifesaving, life-changing, and incredible medicines, it's clear that these companies put their own interests, or the interests of shareholder, ahead of patients.

I spoke to Graham Phillips, registered pharmacist, and owner of multi award-winning iHeart Pharmacy Group. Graham focuses on issues like Type 2 diabetes and cardiovascular disease through his ProLongevity programme.

He's convinced that Big Pharma and Big Food sold the world harmful lies that result in more of these so-called 'lifestyle illnesses':

"Big Food wants us to believe that all calories are the same, which destroys our cardiometabolic health. And then big pharma persuades us to take statins, and lots of other drugs, to kind of palliate."

His research shows that this myth about food is just patently untrue. Our bodies respond differently to different foods, both overall and from person to person. With the ProLongevity programme, people are fitted with blood sugar monitors to show what's causing it to spike.

This promotes both weight loss and helps prevent diabetes by building a clearer picture by looking at a person's individual response to different foods.

Graham recalls fitting a friend with a monitor and seeing a major spike in blood sugar early in the morning. On the call to his friend, he asked what the man had for breakfast. The friend said they'd been eating bran, seeing it as a healthy option. Graham had a different view. He told the man a startling truth, that bran is *high* in sugar. It turns out his All-Bran cereal had 22 grams of sugar per 100 grams. More than Rice Krispies, more than Cheerio's, and twice as much as Corn Flakes. Graham recommended the friend switch to omelettes, which helped the man lose 10 kilos.

Not just that, but it also helped the friend reduce his dependence on medications. You see, the man had high blood pressure and was taking four different medications. On his previous diet, the man's blood pressure was sky high, but thanks to changing his habits the man was able to shrink his medications down to just one.

As Graham points out:

"If you go back 120 years, these diseases simply didn't exist."

If they didn't exist before, there's no reason they should continue to exist. The problem is that there are vested interests in them existing.

After all, when you get down to it, the last thing Big Pharma wants is health. If you think about it, if everyone was healthy then drug makers wouldn't have any customers. They want as many of us to be medicated as possible, and for us to focus on treating problems rather than curing them.

As a healthy man, Graham's friend's life was better, but he was worth less to pharma companies. Stopping all those medications was great for him, but there's no incentive for pharma companies to help us lead healthy lives. Unfortunately, the NHS seems to have sided with Big Pharma too.

The problem with the NHS

Before I say anything else on this, I would like to make the difference between treating acute, critical or specialist conditions—which western medicine is incredible at doing—and lifestyle conditions. The existing medical model works extremely well for what I would call "emergency" situations. The problem we're addressing in this book is that the medical profession has swallowed the lie that lifestyle illnesses are inevitable and that patients will not do what it takes to improve their own health, so a pharmaceutical intervention is the only option in most cases.

They've come to believe that very few patients have the interest or the power to change. In fact, the medical profession seems convinced that all they can do is control people's symptoms, with no ability to address the underlying problems.

As I've mentioned, there's a huge overprescribing problem. I suspect that the underlying cause is that without the time, space and means to really get to the heart a patient's condition, prescribing a medicine to control the symptoms is the only logical thing that can be done.

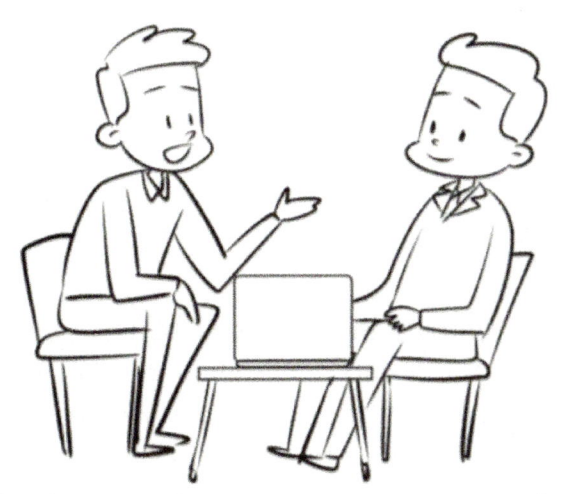

"Right then, we have ten minutes to go through all the factors in your life that maybe making you ill."

It's a problem that benefits pharma companies but should be the opposite of what the NHS aims for. After all, the NHS is meant to be trying to cut down costs to the taxpayer.

Unfortunately, the NHS and Big Pharma are not as separate as most would want them to be. Officials have been accused of taking bribes from pharmaceutical companies to recommend drugs to GPs. Organisations inside the NHS frequently partner with pharma firms in confidential deals.

Perhaps most concerning of all is the fact that the UK's drug regulator, the Medicines and Healthcare products Regulatory Agency (MHRA) is paid for by Big Pharma subscriptions.

Yes, that's right: the drug makers are the ones who fund the drug regulator. No conflict of interest there. If that sounds absurd to you, it's because it is. While the government pays for regulating medical devices, the regulation of medicines is paid for using fees from pharma companies.

Of course, all of that is bad enough on its own, but that's without including another huge flaw with the current system – politics. At this point, the NHS has become a political tool for all sides to wield. They accuse each other of over- or under-spending; of corruption and foul play. Yet in all the talk around the problem, the reality is that politicians are perhaps the last people any of us would want to oversee healthcare.

Their concerns are around re-election and public perception rather than what's necessarily the right thing to do.

==Telling people that they are responsible for their health, that they are the ones with the power, is unpopular.== For that reason, it is seldom ever said. Additionally, politicians typically have little to no experience in the healthcare sector, except as patients. This could make them more susceptible to the lies of Big Pharma when it comes to wellness.

On top of which, politicians can only think short-term. Since there's no guarantee of re-election, it's impossible to plan for more than a few years at a time. This limits the scope of thinking, confining what should be a grand vision for the NHS into these short slivers of time. That leaves no room for long-term planning.

It took a very long time for us to get into the situation we've found ourselves in – where health is getting worse instead of better – and it would likely take a long time for it to get back out again. But nobody at the top can think past the next election date. Worse still, there's this almost perverse incentive not to aim for long-term improvements in case a different political party is in power and takes the credit. With forces like this at work in the world, the situation might seem hopeless. But it's far from it.

First, because, as discussed, our bodies are already well-equipped to heal themselves we have innate support. And secondly, because our lifestyles are also under our control, there's plenty we can do to ease some of the most common long-term conditions.

The NHS is amazing, but it's not the be all and end-all when it comes to our health. Indeed, I have some ideas about how we could improve things...

Chapter 6:
A Better Way for Everyone

"The NHS needs to change fundamentally. Crucially, it doesn't do enough to help people to help themselves."
- Liz Kendall, MP

When Aneurin Bevan first had his vision for the NHS, it was a very different picture from the system we've ended up with. It was understood that social problems such as housing, sanitation, childcare, employment, and cultural factors had a big impact on health.

Before the NHS came into being, Britain's healthcare, and the health of its people, left much to be desired. Officials had recommended that a free national health service should be introduced in England as early as 1920.

However, it wasn't until 1942 and the release of the Beveridge Report, which set out a system of free healthcare funded by taxes, that it seemed possible such an ambitious project could become a reality.

On 6 November 1946 Aneurin 'Nye' Bevan, the Minister of Health in Clement Attlee's Labour government, oversaw the passing of legislation that brought the service into being.

113

In the early days, Bevan faced opposition from doctors who were worried that working for the service would limit their independence and hamstring their income. But he eventually persuaded them to join the NHS, later claiming that he had **'stuffed their mouths with gold.'** He agreed that consultants could keep their private practices and thus retain their financial freedom.

Health was never meant to be about just medicines, but a complete look at how we function as a society. We know that many of the factors we have already discussed all play an important part. But the split between social care and health has been widening ever since. Somewhere along the line we must admit that when it comes to lifestyle conditions, the medical model isn't fit for purpose.

We are now using medicines to try and fix deep societal problems. Of course, this is never going to work.

Sure, we may have taken great strides in controlling symptoms and preventing illnesses getting worse. But we haven't yet mastered the art of improving a patient's quality of life thereafter.

Yet this is exactly what *healing* is all about.

Let doctors do the real work
The current situation with the NHS is just not working. Waiting lists are growing and costs are shooting through the roof. Patients feel powerless,

doctors don't have the time to really make a difference to patients' lives, and the entire system is costing more and more as lifestyle illnesses become more prevalent.

What's needed now is a change in thinking. Not to one that blames and shames people for their bodies, but one that puts patients in charge of their own health. I want doctors to be able to say to patients:

'Look, you have this healing superpower, and you can use it to improve your life, let's work together and help you to unravel your thinking and let's make a plan, then we can add some medicines if we need to help you to achieve your goals.'

This change in approach is happening but I can't see this happening, at scale, anytime soon. However, there is absolutely nothing stopping you from harnessing this power yourself, right now. By learning and understanding the process for creating the placebo effect, you can accelerate your road to complete wellness. You can also use this same skill in other areas of your life too.

When I spoke to Graham about his ProLongevity programme he told me his goal is to eliminate Type 2 diabetes. At first, to me, it sounded incredibly optimistic. But the more I think about it, the more I realise it isn't. These illnesses are new – they don't need to be with us. There's no reason they must be around forever.

And if we could get rid of this illness, and reduce things like obesity and high blood pressure, we could see a radical transformation of the NHS as it stands – one that lets doctors do the work they dreamed of doing.

Without having to deal with so many of these reversible lifestyle illnesses, doctors could spend more time with patients that have very serious health concerns. Wouldn't that be a wonderful outcome?

We know that having a positive experience with a medical professional can be a major contributor to the placebo effect, so imagine how much more effective an appointment would be if you could spend half an hour or more at the GP. Where the GP had the time and space to listen in an empathetic manner and really get to the root of your health concerns.

On top of that, someone might remember in a longer appointment to mention a concerning mole while they are in for an eye infection, possibly detecting a possible skin cancer much earlier on.

Or someone with mental health struggles might feel more comfortable bringing it up after speaking to a doctor about back pain and really being listened to – rather than just pushed out the door with yet another painkiller prescription after less than ten minutes.

Often various differing symptoms could have the same underlying cause. ==This cause could be pathological or a lifestyle choice.== But if we can only discuss one problem per visit what chance is there of getting to these root causes of a patient's problem?

Those of us who have grown up alongside the NHS can hardly imagine our lives without it, and certainly don't want to. Yet the soaring costs and the current state of public health are definite threats, and we need to act if we want to save it. We can't keep writing prescription after prescription for conditions without addressing their root causes and empowering people to go out and fix them.

Whilst we can't wait for the healthcare system to change, or for healthcare practioners to "learn and earn" in a new way, what we can do is take matters into our hands. This is the best way that we can help the NHS and help our doctors to help us. By doing so, we will be actively and genuinely helping to "save the NHS," not just echoing political soundbites.

Our lives are chaotic, and the patterns we've learned in life aren't always our fault. While I do believe we hold responsibility for our lives, I absolutely don't want to blame people for the coping mechanisms they've learned. In many cases, those coping mechanisms were all that they had.

Life is difficult, and it's a mistake to judge others. And for some people it's more difficult than it is for others. (Compassion, empathy and the healing touch must be seen as prerequisites for a person entering the profession not just examination results.)

Once we become aware of these subconscious patterns that affect our lives, I believe it does become our responsibility to find ways of developing new *healthy* patterns of behaviour. Patterns, that not only improve our health, but result in improvements to our very life. This is an opportunity to grow and learn skills that otherwise are low down in the pecking order.

What I want to tell you is that when we are on the right path, we have the power to hold steady and walk it. And when we do, our health will almost certainly start to improve in tangible and meaningful ways.

Right now, you might be in a resting place, a plateau. Maybe you've just had a baby, or lost a loved one, or you're dealing with a major life event. If this is a crisis moment for you, then it might not be possible to do everything I've suggested. But when you are ready, please act. It will change your life.

For those that are ready to move forward but are struggling, I will tell you that you can do what you set out to do. I think we can create a system that supports this approach, which I will go into, but before I do I want to make it clear that this system isn't necessarily the only way for *you* to improve your life. But I am sure it will help.

The truth is, if you are reading this right now, you already have everything you need to succeed in learning how to harness this superpower.

A new way of working
One day I was manning the counter at my old pharmacy and a man came in. The man had just been diagnosed with Type 2 Diabetes, as well as pre-existing hypertension, and brought in a prescription for four different drugs.

I went to hand them over, but he stopped me.
"I want to pay," he said.

"No need," I told him, "Diabetic patients are exempt, so these medicines are free on the NHS for you." He shook his head.

"I want to pay," he repeated. He seemed certain.

Figuring it wasn't worth arguing over, I let him pay for the medicines and leave. Next month comes around, it's the same story. Four medicines for his condition and he insisted on paying once again.

This time I had to ask why he was so dead set on paying when he could get all four for free. He refused to tell me.

Months went by with the exact same pattern. Always the same meds, always the insistence on paying. And while I asked him every time why he wouldn't just take them for free, he wouldn't give me an answer. Until, on month four, the man came in again. Only this time he had no prescriptions.

"Do you need me to check with the doctor?" I asked.

"No, no," he said,

"I'm off all the meds."

Given that he'd refused to explain himself before on any of the previous times he came in, I was half expecting it to stay a mystery forever. This time, though, he was happy to tell me exactly what he'd been up to.

He said that every time he'd had to pay for the medicines, it hurt him. He hated it. But he used it as motivation to exercise and sort out his diet. That got his blood sugar under control, his blood pressure came back into range, and the doctor helped him come off the meds.

For him, the pain of paying for the medicines was greater than the pain of exercising and eating well. And he knew it would be. He set out his plan and he acted on it, and the result was just what he'd been hoping for.

This seems like an incredible example of what could be possible. The decision to pay for prescriptions wouldn't work for everyone, but I think most would agree there needs to be a plan for what to do after diagnosis. A plan that isn't just based on medications but considers the whole person and what they can do to improve their life.

A diagnosis should be the *start* of a journey to make vital improvements to your life, not the end. I absolutely believe doctors should prescribe the needed medications to help control symptoms and stop things getting worse, but we can't keep ending things there. That moment of diagnosis is the time for the patient to start changing perspective and come up with a plan for how to improve their health. Switching from an unhealthy mindset to a healthy one.

That moment is the point where the placebo effect hits its peak – the window where the mind's power to direct healing is at its strongest. If we could just make doctors and patients aware of this opportunity in that crucial moment, it would make such a big difference.

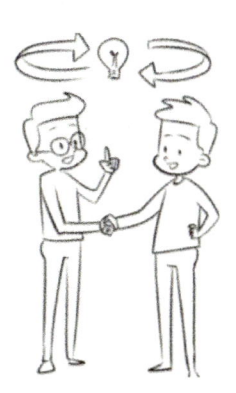

We could direct people to consider a plan that would help them, that addresses their own history and motivations. Maybe they'll come up with a plan like the man I was dealing with at the pharmacy, who went with the stick instead of the carrot.

Or maybe for some people a reward for success works better and they'll promise themselves a weekend away if they can stop smoking.

For too long, we've been focusing exclusively on keeping everyone's heads above water. We can do better. But to do so, the focus needs to be on the person and not the problem.

We need to bring people in and start instigating that moment of change, that shift in focus that can come with a doctor's visit. We can use that moment to activate people, to get them engaged and active in their own health and wellbeing.

Not only that, but we can get people to seriously consider how their health goals intersect with their life goals. It's a moment for reflection and contemplation and stillness.

You might have all heard the famous mindfulness quote by Jon Kabat Zinn:

'You can't stop the waves. But you can learn to surf.'

This quote provides us with a wonderful picture of the road ahead. If the NHS could see this for the opportunity it really is, that each therapeutic encounter with the medical system is a moment where we could be working to cultivate the placebo effect, the potential is enormous. This is the very foundation for triggering the healing process.

Importantly, the emphasis would be on our own power. Our own ability to succeed at our health goals if we open ourselves up to change. In an ideal NHS, doctors and patients would work together, but with an emphasis on our own ability to work towards wellness.

The current system almost imagines the doctor as the mechanic and the patient as a car in need of repair. Instead, we should be encouraged to see each other as equals, as human beings. We all have challenges in life that we have to navigate through, some of us are better at it than others, however we all have the capacity to learn better coping mechanisms and increase our resilience.

The doctor might be able to diagnose the problem, but wellness requires effort on both sides. We are not passive; we are active agents in our own care. I would love to see this attitude permeate throughout the NHS, and even worldwide, there are various initiatives and pilots that show this approach has merit but has a long way to go for grassroots implementation.

Until then, I'll tell you this:

You can recognise your own ability to achieve your health goals and you can choose to embrace the steps behind the placebo effect. ==You don't need anybody else for that.== You can start today by harnessing your own innate superpower, by harnessing the power of the placebo effect. Your life deserves this.

Chapter Seven:
There's nothing stopping you from evolving

"The decisive moment in human evolution is perpetual."
- Franz Kafka

When I first started coaching Mary, she was eighteen. She was extremely organised, and I don't just mean for her age. She already had a five-year plan before even leaving college. She was incredibly smart too, getting straight As. You could just tell she had incredible potential.

Early on, I asked her what she wanted to do, and she said she wanted to be a teacher. When she told me, I tried not to show my concern. I knew right away it was a bad fit. If she'd been my teacher in school, Mary would probably have gone home crying every day. Her kind, innocent and gentle nature was not suited to the current environment in our schools.

Teaching is one of the most intense jobs out there. I'd put it up there with paramedics and firefighters in terms of the toll it can take on people. Children can experience all sorts of childhood trauma and be subjected to neglect or abuse, and teachers are frequently on the front lines of that. They often bear the brunt of a child's frustration.

A study by teachers' union NASUWT showed that one in four teachers were subject to weekly physical attacks from pupils. It takes a tough skin to survive in education, but Mary didn't have that, yet. I could see how the job would wear her down bit by bit.

It seemed to me like Mary had decided to be a teacher without stopping to think if it was really a good fit. However, I didn't want to go straight in and crush her dreams. Instead, I started by asking why she wanted to be a teacher. It turned out that Mary's mum was a teaching assistant, which may have planted the idea of teaching in her mind.

So, I decided to work on expanding her way of thinking, stressing that she might want to push herself beyond the more stable career path she'd imagined. At 18, did she really need to push for a twenty- or thirty-year career when she didn't know yet if it would work out? Had she thought more seriously about her options?

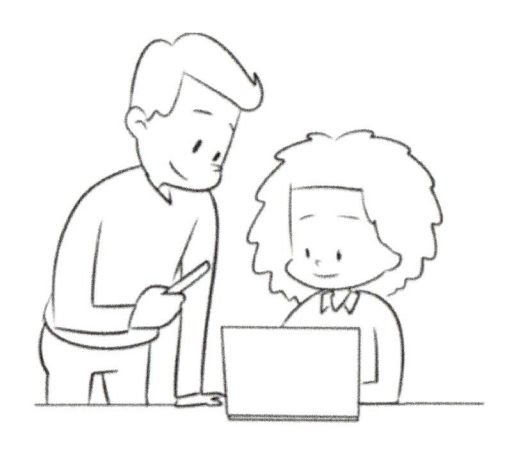

In the process, we both began to see the block she had against considering other careers. Teaching was a 'safe' job in her mind, but she started to realise that she wasn't looking for something safe just yet. She was young, smart and driven and started to embrace the idea of adventure in her life.

With this shift in perspective, she's found herself in several vibrant and exciting careers. She worked for Sky News, BBC, she won a contest to become the face of Intu, became a UN ambassador, and is now one of the BBC's youngest ever assistant producers.

In fact, she's been able to fulfil her teaching role in a new way as she works on children's education channel CBeebies Bite Size.

Teaching is obviously a tremendous gift to the world, and one of the most valuable things a person could be, but the Mary of today would be a far better teacher than the young woman I met at eighteen. She has real life successes and experience.

If she'd stuck to the path she was on before, none of that would have happened for her. Most likely she'd have been frustrated and exhausted, burned out before she'd even started in life.

On the surface, Mary's story doesn't look like it's about health at all, but it is. It's about the kind of health I think we should all strive for.

We need to make sure that the paths we choose will keep us healthy – not just physically, but mentally too. I won't pretend that means there are any easy choices. But when we can, we should check that those are our choices, coming from within, not the choices of our family or society.

We often start trying to climb the ladder without first checking it's leaning against the right wall. We climb aimlessly, one rung after the other, often trying not to look at the other ladders going to places we wish we could. Then, if we find we've chosen wrong, we must climb down from where we are and back up a different ladder.

How often do we hear about people who reach their goals and are still unsatisfied? No wonder we make ourselves sick with work.

When we're on the wrong path our motivation is non-existent, and we feel like we're wading through mud to get anywhere, while other people move forward effortlessly around us.

Understanding yourself
A crucial aspect of health is that it's personal to each of us. What's healthy in one person's life might seem chaotic in somebody else's, and even then, it can change over time. Mary wasn't at the right point in life at eighteen to decide to become a teacher, but there are others who'd be perfectly suited to it then.

Unfortunately, many of us are not as in tune with ourselves as we'd like to be. Mary wanted to follow in her mother's footsteps and meet family expectations. Like many of us, she'd been led by the messages around her that it was secure work, it's a good job. But she had more going for her but never had the opportunity to explore.

We have all these voices coming from the outside telling us what we should do, that we should find a partner; we should have children; we should stick to a safe career. With all these voices echoing around in our minds, it's no wonder we struggle to hear our own inner voice.

That inner voice can be drowned out, but it can't be silenced. By stifling and avoiding it, we make ourselves sick. Ignoring the voice that tells us this is the wrong career, the wrong partner, the wrong time for children, is absolutely exhausting. It's a full-time job trying to cover it up. We try everything from drugs and alcohol to mindless scrolling through social media, anything that makes the voice as quiet as possible, so we don't have to listen to it. That way we don't have to realise we've made a mistake.

How can we become healthy when we act like that? How, if we are trying to make our own inner light as dim as possible, can we ever get well?
We can't. It's as simple as that. We can't.

==So, if we *want* to be well, we need to quiet all the other voices down until we can hear ourselves think.== Health requires self-knowledge. I would go so far as to say that it might be impossible to reach a true state of relaxation if we are afraid of what our minds have to say. Otherwise, each time we take time to ourselves to be still and quiet, the thoughts that come to us just stress us out more.

If you want to be well, you need to get to know your body too. You can also learn how your body responds to some foods versus others, or to different kinds of exercise. Maybe running hurts your knees but swimming is much easier.

We can build positive habits and lifestyle choices that suit us personally. By doing so, not only will we get healthier, but we will be happier doing these things.

In fact, let's have a look at the 'Flow' diagram again and see what happens if we add Maslow's Hierarchy of Needs to this picture.

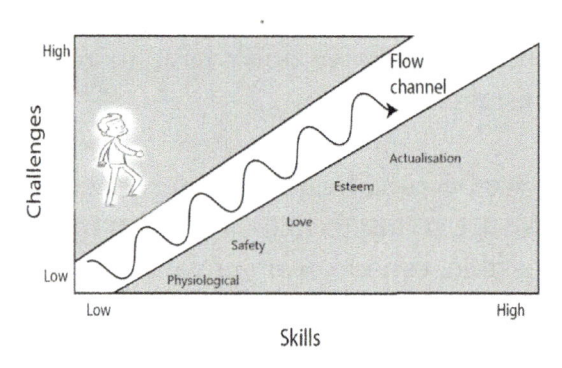

Does this start to make a bit more sense, now? This is the journey we all must take.

You build an understanding of how your mind and body work together. You understand the importance of getting the mind and body in sync. Maybe you are unhappy with your job and it's driving you to snack more or smoke more at work to stave off the boredom. Maybe you and your partner are going through a difficult time, and the stress is causing digestion or sleep problems.

Knowing doesn't mean things have to change right away, or at all. Perhaps you dislike your job, but it allows you to stay in a beloved community and the trade-off is worth it for you. Maybe the current situation is almost over, and things will improve soon. The key learning is being conscious and aware so that you can adapt and act when the opportunity arises.

Knowledge and insights that we've been keeping from ourselves have the power to unlock something deep inside us and can make things so much better.

Once we know ourselves, we can use that knowledge. We can decide if a job is working or not. We can decide if our current trajectory is in line with our goals. There are always choices, whether we're reaching the height of a career or facing the end of life. We can decide to leave a toxic situation.

Or we can learn more skills and increase our ability to cope and thrive through life's challenges, rather than merely surviving them.

When we're open to thinking critically about the direction we're going in, we're ready to start listening to our inner voice. That inner voice is intelligent and intuitive.

When we listen to that voice, then we can use it to shape our lives and grow as people. And when we control our life, we can choose to prioritise our health.

The importance of a tangible benefit

Just as there are all kinds of forces pushing us down the wrong path, we may have a fight on our hands trying to turn back.

The current that carried us so smoothly in the wrong direction becomes a riptide when we try to swim against it. We can lose valued relationships or create conflict with family and friends seemingly out of nowhere.

The people who surround us are not always happy when we succeed. I think this is something in human nature we hate to admit to. Think about the backlash singer Adele received for losing weight. When we change, the people around us don't always support us like we'd hoped. Instead, they try to force us back into the people we used to be.

Maybe it makes them feel more comfortable to see others doing the same thing. People are resistant to change, especially in the people around them. When we decide to grow, the people who are leaning on us for support can start to feel unstable.

They get worried we won't be there for them anymore. On top of that, when we make a change, other people can seem to take offence. It's as if they take *our* decisions as a criticism of *their* actions. If you try to cut down on your drinking, others might get annoyed because it feels like you're judging them for continuing.

Most likely you're just thinking that you'd rather not have a hangover on the weekend, but to everyone else you've become an annoying goody two shoes, ruining the fun. So, if we want to be healthy, we must actually… *want to be healthy*.

We must decide that all the trouble is worth it. If we might lose friends, or get mocked by co-workers, we'd better have a good reason to keep going. We must know how the changes we make for our health line up with our other goals.

When Mary first decided against teaching and started to assess her other options, once she stepped out of her comfort zone, she found that she was much more in demand than she'd ever thought. As she said yes to more and more new career opportunities, offers started coming in all the time.

Her struggle at that point was figuring out which of these opportunities truly aligned with her ambitions, and which didn't.

She'd figured out more about herself, she was listening to her own inner voice for guidance, but she still had decisions to make. Should she take this or that job when both appealed for different reasons? Should she relocate for a passion project, or stay closer to home with a still exciting opportunity?

Questions like this seem reasonable but can be a path away from wellness. We need some method to sort out what will or won't work for us. For that, we need to keep an eye on our ultimate goals.

These are the kind of big picture ideas about life that few of us have much time to think about. It's not enough to just listen to our own inner voice, we must let that voice shine through in our lives. The inner voice is abstract, it wants or does not want things. It's our job to make that into a reality.

If my inner voice tells me I am exhausted with my job, that's just the start of a bigger journey. I need to decide what to do about it: maybe I have taken on too much, or I'm feeling undervalued, or I need to change careers entirely.

When we are aiming for a healthy life, it needs to be visible in our actions. It needs to be part of our goals. When we make decisions about our future, our health concerns need to be part of the decision-making process at all times. Maybe we're offered an opportunity with an exciting-looking job, but the corporate culture involves heavy drinking every week. When health isn't on our radar, it's possible to imagine taking the job and disregarding the impact of alcohol on our health.

However, if health has become a fixed part of how we imagine our future, then such a job would be unthinkable. Because we want a healthy life, and we're unwilling to let anything get in the way of that.

This is part of the placebo effect too, this incredible boost that can come from making our health goals into life goals, the desire and expectation to live well.

Where it wouldn't even occur to us to make choices that deliberately sacrifice our wellbeing for the sake of money, or status, or even relationships.

What's more, health can reward us in ways nothing else can. When we give ourselves more strength, more power, more flexibility…our brains release all sorts of chemicals in response that improve our overall mood, making our lives richer and more fulfilling.

135

Conclusion:
How The Placebo Effect can help you take control of your own health

"Change, before you have too."
— *Jack Welch*

As I explained in this book, we can breakdown our understanding of how the placebo effect could be harnessed consciously into three distinct stages.

In fact, I believe we can turn these stages into steps that you can follow to help unlock the healing power of the placebo effect for yourself, whether you do so with or without medication.

In this final part of the book, I'd like to go through each of these steps to show how you might use them in your own life to help put in place the platform you need to make healthier choices.

Step One: Achieving a state of deep relaxation
We all have the capacity to heal ourselves. Beyond just cuts and scrapes, the trillions of cells in our bodies are constantly dying and being replaced with new cells. Our bodies can generate a whole new upper layer of skin in just 28 days, new lungs in about six weeks. All of us are in a constant state of repair and rejuvenation.

Estimates suggest that as much as 98% of the cells in your body change every year. That means the body you are sitting is almost all brand new. It's not the same body that sat here last year, and it won't be the same next year either. So, if the body completely regenerates, why does illness stay year in and year out? Well, maybe we're not giving our bodies a chance to heal.

Scientifically, it all comes down to the autonomic nervous system, a system in the body that controls unconscious functions like digestion, breathing, heart rate, and so on. This system has two divisions: the sympathetic and parasympathetic nervous systems. The two systems work in opposition to each other.

The parasympathetic is active when the body and mind are in a state of relaxation and repair, what's sometimes called the "rest or digest" function (the opposite of fight/flight). It's only in this state, when we're relaxed, that our bodies are truly primed to regenerate.

Meanwhile, the sympathetic activates when we enter fight/flight mode. It prepares us for danger and focuses only on the core functions we need to survive. Once we're exposed to something stressful, our bodies release a cascade of hormones like cortisol and adrenaline that spike blood pressure and make our hearts beat faster. Breathing changes, and so do insulin levels, as we gear ourselves up to deal with the threat.

Unfortunately, this state comes at the expense of many other important functions. You see, our stress response evolved to handle intense life-or-death situations like sudden attacks from sabre-toothed tigers. It's supposed to be a temporary state, one that passes once we're out of danger.

This is where the story of our chronic health struggles really starts to make sense. What happens if you're in that 'fight/flight' state all day long but without any real danger?

Worryingly, there's a growing body of evidence showing how, in modern society, many of us are now living in a state of mild fight/flight. Even though nothing life-threatening is happening, we're still stressed. It turns out there doesn't need to be any real danger for fight/flight response to kick in: we can activate it ourselves with our own fears, whether they are rational or not.

As we go around worrying about our families, our friends, our jobs, we keep switching on that sympathetic system and switching off our healing system. We even do things that seem designed to stress us out – watching depressing news stories about the economy, natural disasters, conflicts.

Five hundred years ago, Michel de Montaigne said:

"My life has been filled with terrible misfortune; most of which never happened."

There's even a study that proves it. It turns out that 85 percent of the things people worried about never actually happened.

What's more, our bodies don't know the difference between a real imminent danger and an imagined one. Whether the stress comes from the mind or from something stalking towards us with sharp claws, it's the same system that's activated. Although, this is not always to the same extent. On top of that, we get so used to these chronic stresses that we start to see them as simply part of life, inevitable and unavoidable.

The common approach of just allowing our worries to take hold may be harmful. Many studies have found that as much as 80% of patients reported uncommon emotional stress before their disease began. Worse still, not only does stress cause disease, but the disease itself then stresses us out even more, creating a vicious cycle.

We can't always be in a relaxed state and stress can be helpful on some occasions. When we're learning and growing, stress can be an important part of that cycle. All life inevitably comes with stresses, ranging from trivial traffic jams to major events like bereavements. These not only tax the mind, but the body as well.

Another complication is that our bodies can become stressed without us even knowing. Think about how much harder the body must work when we're eating the wrong kinds of foods, or when it must remove the toxins from drinking and smoking. These constant challenges to the body start to wear us down over time. It's like driving to a petrol station and putting diesel into your petrol engine. How long would the car drive before the engine gave up and needed to go the garage for repair?

By punishing our bodies in this way, we keep ourselves in that constant stress mode, the sympathetic system is always on while our systems for rest and repair are switched off.

So, the question arises, when do we give ourselves time and space to repair, rejuvenate, and replace our cells? When do we regain the space in our minds that has been hijacked by stresses and fears? Most which may never even happen. But the fear can leave us in a state of growth paralysis and stagnation or leave us totally overwhelmed with our lives.

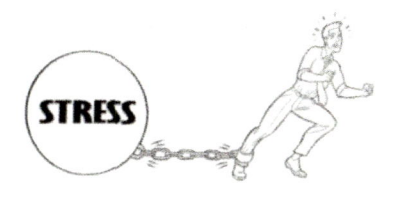

"Is the stress in your life holding you back?"

Here's a quick test. Take a deep breath. Notice where you were breathing from.

Was it a deep belly diaphragm breath or was it your upper chest region that moved the most? If it was the latter, you could well be experiencing some degree of fight/flight response.

Now take a moment to sense where there is stress or tension in your body. Do you have tight shoulders? Back pain? These are all indicators that you may be operating from the sympathetic nervous system (fight/flight mode) rather than the parasympathetic nervous system (rejuvenation mode - homoeostasis).

If you're living this way, tense and always on guard, it stacks the odds of good health against you. Living with the sympathetic system always at the wheel gives our bodies very little time for rest or repair.

Luckily, it turns out that reversing this is key part of how the placebo effect works. We can reclaim the space that stress takes up in our minds and life. Now, if you can do that exercise again but this time consciously breath slower. Focus on relaxing and deepening your breathing. You can, now, focus on those areas where there is tension and imagine the tension dissolving away.

This is simple technique where you can start to experience what is possible. If you did this 'reset' every day for about 15-20 mins the benefits to health, clarity of decision making, and performance will be tangible and positive.

Imagine you are sitting in a doctor's office. You've been stressed for days about your symptoms. Maybe you've been looking around online and getting some frightening search results back, making you even more nervous. Your sympathetic nervous system is firing on full cylinders. Fear and anxiety take hold.

When you do finally see the doctor, she is kind and patient. She takes careful note of your symptoms and listens to your concerns. You trust her opinion. She sends you for a test and you leave her office confident in her ability to get to the bottom of things and figure it all out.

This reassurance helps you to accept the situation and allows the fight/flight system to switch off. The immediate threat has disappeared. It is now manageable. A shift in mindset has occurred.

We can see how easy a mindset can shift when a person has time and space to process things in the right manner. Often this can happen spontaneously as the person is unravelling. Insights, solutions, a sense of 'knowing' the right thing to do, all arise into a person's awareness.

At the same time, we know that there is an increase of helpful and healing hormones, chemicals and neurotransmitters that enhance these feelings of wellness (albeit temporary) whilst at the same time a decrease in stress hormones such as cortisol. A cascade of these internal physical changes works *synergistically* with the internal mental changes to prepare you for the healing process ahead.

Now, the appointment is over. You may know deep down that you've needed to change things for a while, but never had the strength or motivation, or even the opportunity. This therapeutic intervention gives a brief moment for reflection. You see that there is no other choice. Something must give.

This you know isn't really a bad thing, as these changes are long overdue. You mull them over in your head. You start to rationalise your situation and as you begin to see the light at the end of the tunnel, that worry you've been carrying around leading up to seeing the doctor is gone. You head home feeling lighter, sure that your care is in good hands. You accept the situation, knowing you'll get through this and get better.

This, in my experience, is the first stage of the placebo effect. It's subtle but powerful. Before you went to the doctor there's a good chance that your body was in fight/flight mode, fear of diagnosis, effect of symptoms on your life. Possibly stifling your ability to heal. During the appointment, being reassured, having trust in the doctor, being listened too and having your concerns taken seriously all have an internal subconscious effect, you entered the relaxed and open state of mind that allows healing to take place. No treatment was received at this point, just the ability to switch that stress response off and feel calm once again.

You reset.

It's crucial to realise that this ability to reset and shift your mindset, to settle the body back into its natural parasympathetic state, is always available to us. The ability to do this, consciously and at will, is our superpower. As Bruce Lee said:

"One of the best things that you can learn is to master how to stay calm. Calm is a superpower."

We can choose to enter this restful rejuvenation state, to take time for some form of focused relaxation, and increase our own capacity to heal ourselves.

Step Two: Activating Your Natural Lifeforce
Our lifeforce is the most intelligent, sensitive, creative, and powerful substance known to man. It's also the least understood.

It's suggested that our lifeforce, our innate intelligence, is responsible for everything from remembering to breathe and keeping your heart pumping, to understanding and solving complex equations. It is also responsible for our healing, repair, and rejuvenation.

Our lifeforce directs growth from two single cells into the trillions of cells, which make the skin, muscles, brain, bones, eyes, the capacity to think, feel, smell, taste, and even to reason. Everything you experience, do and think is all done with and by this life force.

When we can build up this lifeforce—as we can attempt to in Tai chi and Yoga—individuals experience heightened feelings of wellbeing. They feel more energetic, experience a greater clarity in thinking and enjoy a better quality of sleep.

This increase in lifeforce can be the source of the extra energy you need to educate yourself about you and your condition. Maybe as some traditions suggest, this lifeforce is the healing power itself.

Let's imagine, once again, that a person is in the consultation room of his healthcare professional…

He is feeling a little stressed but in generally feels fine. A routine check shows high blood pressure. While this isn't life threatening right now, chronic high blood pressure could have serious complications long-term if it's not controlled. The doctor asks if he is getting enough rest or if there is any stress in life. His mind starts to throw up all sorts of stressful situations that he has had to endure lately. The demands of his job, conflict with a loved one, a child making poor life decisions, debts piling up.

He begins to see how all these little stresses niggle away at his peace of mind. The internal process has begun. The old, unhealthy mindset is being challenged.

She suggests taking a break from work if he can, and stresses how important it is to be getting a good night's sleep. She also asks about exercise, explaining that it can help to work out stress and build resilience. Before arriving at the doctors' office, he had regularly been staying up much too late, burning the candle at both ends. The workplace has a 'work hard, play hard' mentality, but the combination of long hours and heavy drinking are wearing him down.

This revelation from a calm and competent medical professional puts thing in a different perspective. The shock of the diagnosis unsettles. But he is open to change, even for that split second. He trusts their experience. He soon realises that there could be other areas of his life that are suffering and so thinks seriously about making a change. Something inside him gets 'activated'. He has become motivated to improve his health, taking on the responsibility of bringing his blood pressure to a healthy level. Almost immediately, he is shifting the odds in his own favour.

This is what I mean by activation. Something inside you changes and the energy you need for change is freed. You might start looking for a new job, or studying more, or even find the strength to leave a toxic relationship. The repetitive patterns that you were living on repeat stop being subconscious habits, letting you decide what to keep and what to get rid of. Activation is essentially an educational experience.

Researchers in psychedelics have found that when we break the loop of negative thinking, the brain starts communicating within itself better. This can give people access to more mind power in the decision-making process, helping them to make better life choices.

The result is a feeling of wellness as the mind reconnects and works in a more wholesome manner. Healing, after all, comes from the word whole. Relaxation and activation can reset you and make you whole, temporarily, but the final challenge is to keep up healthy changes long-term.

Step Three: Build Self-Care into Your Life
Did you know that patients who engaged in selfcare/self-management practices have been shown to reduce the burden on the NHS by as much as 80%?

We have the awareness that we should care more about our health. Most of us we know we should eat better and exercise more. But it's hard to bring that knowledge in line with our other goals. This aspect is complicated, and difficult, but this is the key to long lasting health and a good quality of life. It ultimately comes down to the way we act day-to-day. Our family, our culture, and or our environment all shape the way we think and behave. The ancient Greek physician who created the Hippocratic Oath, Hippocrates, shared many profound insights into healing, but the one that's most apt here is:

"Before you heal someone, ask him if he is willing to give up the things that made him sick."

Just take a moment and think about that.

Hippocrates was born thousands of years ago, living in a world almost completely unlike the one we're in today. And yet, this fundamental truth, that we as humans often cling to the things that make us ill, has not changed.

We think and act in certain ways because we're expected to, or out of habit, without regard to whether it's what's best for us. Psychologists currently believe most of our decision-making processes are unconscious. We think we are in control of our lives, but our upbringing, our education, our society, and the impressions these make on our minds are the most important factors.

Freud says time and time again: *we are puppets of the subconscious.* Perhaps we know that we should go to bed earlier, but we're stuck in a loop of watching TV until late into the evening before scrolling through our phones well past midnight.

Eventually, these bad habits carve deep tracks in our minds like water wearing through rock. We find ourselves returning to these thoughts all the time, reinforcing them over and over until they feel inescapable. Our thoughts and actions become automatic as they run through the grooves, grooves we have created in ourselves. What if we consciously made new grooves that allowed life to flow in a much healthier, wholesome and rewarding way? Making new grooves (new habits and ways of thinking) is a process that many don't have the time or energy for.

F.M Alexander, the founder of the 'Alexander Technique' once said:

"People don't decide their future, they decide their habits and their habits decide the future."

If we want to change, we need to take a proactive approach to our lives. I believe this is the final piece of the puzzle when it comes to the placebo effect: we must accept and pick up the burden of our own health. The struggles and pains, the criticism from friends and family, the time sacrificed for exercise or meditation.

I know that this is a painful burden to shoulder, and one that our childhood does almost nothing to prepare us for. We're sent out into the world with vague knowledge of academic subjects – maths, history, physics – and whatever habits (good or bad) we've picked up from the people around us.

Plus, unlike with work or education, there are almost no teachers around us. There's little education around healthy eating and exercise, except maybe a few minutes looking at the food pyramid (designed by the industry, by the way). Adding to that, we're bombarded day and night by people and companies who are trying to make us consume more and more.

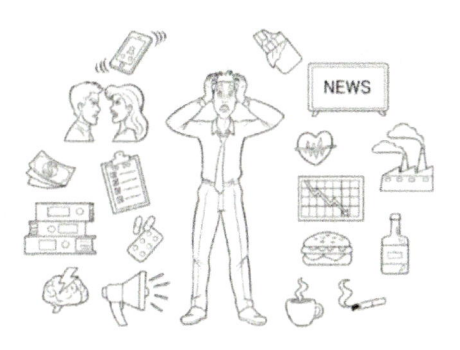

Giant companies are trying to sell us more electronics and media that keep us inside, make us eat more processed foods, drink more alcohol, read books on fad diets, this diet, that diet, and take stacks of different medications. They don't care if we are well. In fact, many of these businesses would prefer it if we weren't.

When we hear a phrase like 'taking responsibility,' it often feels hollow. There's rarely any empathy in it. Something goes wrong, and rather than compassion we're told to take responsibility. It's said as though it's effortless, as though corporations aren't spending billions upon billions trying to make us sick and keep us that way.

By the time people showed up in my pharmacy they were often exhausted. Disease rarely comes on overnight, and the processes that get us to that point are rarely simple.

So, I want to take a moment to acknowledge that what I'm advocating for in this book is not a "quick fix". The health problems each of us face are not straightforward, and they don't have simple answers.

Self-Care can be exhausting and difficult. I think it's cruel to pretend otherwise. Lifestyle changes are hard. Therapy is hard. Meditation and yoga are hard. Giving up coping mechanisms is hard. More to the point life can be hard. However, the most important thing to remember is that growth and change are worth it, and also inevitable.

When I say we must be responsible for our own health, I understand that what I'm suggesting can be difficult. The truth is that life can be hard at times. It does require us to keep growing, to keep learning, adapting. But once we accept this, we can stop fighting against it, stop running away from it, and we can find the strength to rise to the challenge.

No matter how you might feel, it's far from a hopeless situation. Even when nobody else is on our side, we can be.

152

To help, I propose incorporating a new 'five-a-day' into your life. The current idea that eating five pieces of fruit or vegetables is enough to keep you healthy and happy just doesn't work. It's only a small part of looking after yourself. Instead, I believe your 'five-a-day' should be thought about like this:

1. **Good Nutrition**
    a. Protein
    b. Low carbs/low sugar
    c. Hydration

2. **Regular Movement**
    a. Aerobic
    b. Stretch
    c. Resistance training

3. **Deep Rest**
    a. Relaxation
    b. Reset

4. **Social Activity**
    a. Hobbies
    b. Social life
    c. Loving Relationships

5. **Purpose**
    a. Meaningful work
    b. Exploring potential

We can be our own advocates, choosing to stand up for the health of our minds and our bodies.

We can work to understand ourselves and make it our mission to improve our own lives. We can learn about our health conditions, how to manage them, and what works for us. Studies of self-care show that it's an incredibly effective tool. We keep finding evidence of self-care's effectiveness across a wide range of conditions such as asthma, depression, diabetes, heart disease, arthritis, and chronic pain.

What's more, evidence shows that managing our own health can have enormous benefits. As you know there is ample evidence that self-management courses could cut down on visits to health professionals by as much as 80%. Yes, 80%.

Plus, a study in the US found that self-management programmes boosted health status and cut down emergency department visits. This approach can also reduce pain, boost quality of life, and help reduce the severity of symptoms.

These programmes typically involve learning about our own health conditions, how to manage them, and how to seek support. These are all questions we can answer for ourselves with time and patience.

We can go a step further and think about how an illness affects us specifically. We can pay attention to easing the symptoms we do have, in a preventative manner, and how our own bodies respond to different treatments. We can pay attention to how food, exercise, weather, mood, and many other factors interact with our bodies. It's a way to express appreciation for ourselves, and to treat ourselves better.

Your body is a marvellous machine. Self-repairing, self-healing, and capable of sometimes miraculous things. Through our bodies we can experience everything life has to offer us. By helping our bodies, instead of harming them, we can make our days more joyful, more beautiful.

With self-care, we have the full power of the placebo effect on our side. I choose to believe the existence of this effect is evidence of our own power to be well.

When we are calm, and active, and looking after ourselves, we can achieve so much more than we might have thought possible. We can cultivate within ourselves a sense of tranquillity and purpose. We can have compassion for ourselves throughout life's challenges, and we can find the determination to overcome them.

This is the Power of The Placebo Effect.

This is Our Innate Superpower.

Our Secret Superpower.

If you would like to speak to me about anything in this book, would like to book a wellbeing consultation, or you want to find out about our other incredible products, feel free to email me

enquiries@psy-qi.com

Highlights from the Research

There are 17 million people in the UK suffering from long term conditions that is **1 in 2 adults** (NHS Confederation Conference 2007).

Instigating a self-management programme has been shown to reduce **follow up visits to general practitioners by up to two fifths.**

Self-management courses may **reduce visits to all health professionals by up to 80%.**

1 in 4 people will experience some kind of mental health problem in the course of a year. 1 in 6 people are experiencing this right now. (Office for National Statistics Psychiatric Morbidity Report 2001)

Work related stress, depression or anxiety alone accounted for an estimated **13.5 million lost working days** in Britain in one year. (Labour Force Survey 2008)

In 1999, The Independent on Sunday in the United Kingdom estimated that **more than 30,000 people in Britain were addicted to painkillers.** Such mishandled drugs now kill 20,000 a year, nearly twice as many as 10 years ago.

For one in 10 people in the UK, anxiety interferes with normal life. Excessive anxiety is often associated with other mental health problems, such as depression. Anxiety is only considered to be a mental health problem when it's long lasting, severe and is interfering with everyday activities.

According to a recent World Mental Health Survey, generalised anxiety disorder, or Gad (that is, constant worrying about all the things that might go wrong), has become the most prevalent mental-health problem in the world — creating an "anxiety epidemic"

A community based self-management programme involving 551 people with heart disease, lung disease or type 2 diabetes, showed participants had better health status, health behaviour, and self-efficacy **and fewer emergency department visits** compared to those receiving usual care. These improvements were maintained after one year.

A review of self-management programmes showed a tendency for people to report reduced severity of symptoms and pain, and improved life control, activity, resourcefulness, and life satisfaction.

Diabetics showed a clear improvement in quality of life. But this effect took a long time to develop **but was still present at four years.**

Self-management can work for everyone. A study from 2004 showed self-management improved satisfaction with care in a cognitively impaired group.

A UK based randomised study over five years involving over 100 patients showed that chronic disease self-management programmes were associated with **improved healthy behaviours,** coping, communication with physicians, **self-reported health status and reduced days in hospital.**

A self-management programme in Hong Kong showed **reduced hospitalisations and reduced the length of hospital stay by up to half.**

A review of self-management in the Lancet showed 57% of self-management intervention programmes showed improvements in lung function. **It also concluded that stress and emotions management** as well as behaviour can be successful in improving lung function in asthma.

Self-management education **reduced hospital re-admissions threefold** for adults with asthma.

In a community self-management programme involving people with heart disease, lung disease or type 2 diabetes, it was shown that participants had **better health status, health behaviour, and self-efficacy and fewer accident and emergency**

department visits compared to those receiving usual care.

A home based cognitive-behavioural, self-management rehabilitation programme for myocardial infarction patients **reduced re-admissions by 30%**

A randomised trial showed that participants in three sessions of self-management education on heart failure who then adopted self-management strategies were at **lower risk of death and readmission to hospital.**

Further reading

Choosing health. Making healthy choices easier. Nov 2004.

Dawn of a new era for pharmacy. 2005.

Integrating the NHS. The NHS handbook 1999.

The need for a new medical model. A Challenge for Biomedicine. Science 1977.

Self-Care Conference report 2013.

The Case for Investing in Self-Care May13.

Helping People Help Themselves.

A Practical Guide To Self Management Support.

The Okinawa Way: a 25-year study on health

Perfect Health. Dr Deepak chopra.

You are the Placebo. Dr Joe Dispenza

Doctor You. Jeremy Horwick

Why Woo-Woo Works. David Hamilton Ph. D

The PolyVagal Theory. Stephen Porges.

NLP and Health. O'Connor, J. McDermott.I.

Promoting Health: a practical guide. 4th edition
Ewles L, Simnett I 1999

Health promotion through self-care and community participation: elements of a proposed programme in the developing countries. BMC public health. Bhuyan.K. K (2004)

Psychoneuroimmunology finds acceptance as science adds evidence. The scientist. Benowitz (1996).

Psychological stress and the human immune system: A meta-analytical study of 30 years of inquiry. Psychological bulletin, vol 130 4. Segerstrom. S & Miller.G

The Relaxation Response. Herbert Benson. (1975)

Psychoneuroimmunology: Can psychological interventions modulate immunity? Jornal of consulting and clinical psychology Vol 60 4. Kiecolt-Glaser. J.K & Glaser. R (1992)

Use of Mind-Body Therapies. Journal of internal medicine. Vol 19 1. wolsko.P.M, Eisenberg.D.M, Davies, R.B, Phillips.R. S (2004)
Psychoneuroimmunology and health psychology: An Integrative model. Brain, Behavior and immunity. 17. Lutgendorf.S. K Costanzo.E. S (2003)

Consciousness and Healing. University of Arizona College of Medicine. Weil.A. T

Psychological factors and Psychoneuroimmunology within a lifespan perspective. Development of health and the wealth of nations: social, biological and educational dynamics. Coe. C. L. (1999)

Enhancing Human Healing. BMJ. Reilly. D. (2001)

Expectancy, therapeutic instructions and the placebo response. Placebo: theory research and mechanism. Evans, F.

Lorig KR, Mazonson PD, Homan HR. Evidence suggesting that health education for self-management in patients with chronic arthritis has sustained health benefits while reducing health care costs. Arth Rheum 1993; 36(4): 439-46

Fries JF, Carey C Mc Shane DJ. Patient education in arthritis: randomized controlled trial of mail-delivered program. J Rheumatology 1997; 24(7): `378-83

Groessl EJ, Cronan TA. A cost analysis of Self-management programs for people with chronic illness. Am J Comm Psy 2000; 28(4): 455-80

Barlow JH et al. Self management literature review. Psychosocial Research Centre, Coventry University, 2000

Trente M, Passera P et al. lifestyle intervention by group care prevents deterioration of type II diabetes: a 4years randomized controlled clinical trial. Diabetologia 2002; 45: 1231 -39

Schiel R, Braun A, Muller R, et al. A structured treatment and education program for patients with type 2 diabetes mellitus, insulin therapy and impaired cognitive function (Dikol). Med Klin 2004; 99(6):285-92

Newman S, Steed L, Mulligan K. Self-management interventions for chronic illness. The Lancet. Oct 23-29, 2004. Vol. 364, Iss 9444; pg 1523-1538.

Warsi A, Wang PS, laValley MP, et al. Self-management education programs in chronic disease: a systemic review and methodological critique of the literature. Arch Intern Med 2004; 164(15): 1641-9

The British liver Trust. Living a healthy Life with Long Term Illness. Leland Stanford Junior University 1999

Newman S, Steed L, Mulligan K. Self-management interventions for chronic illness. The Lancet. Oct 23-29, 2004. Vol. 364, Iss 9444; pg 1523-1538.

Lorig KR, Ritter PL, Gonzalez VM. Hispanic chronic disease Self-management: a randomized communitybased outcome trial. Nurs Res 2003; 52(6):361-9 6/52

Lefort SM. A test of Braden's Self-Help Model in adults with chronic pain. J Nursing Scholarship 2000; 32(2):153-60

Wright SP, Walsh H, Ingley KM et al. Uptake of Self-management strategies in a heart failure management programme. Eur J Heart Fail 2003; 5(3): 371-80

Printed in Great Britain
by Amazon